The Practice of Electroconvulsive Therapy: Recommendations for Treatment, Training, and Privileging

**The American Psychiatric Association
Task Force on Electroconvulsive Therapy**

Richard D. Weiner, M.D., Ph.D. *(Chairperson)*
Max Fink, M.D.
Donald W. Hammersley, M.D.
Iver F. Small, M.D.
Louis A. Moench, M.D.
Harold Sackeim, Ph.D. *(Consultant)*

APA Staff

Harold Alan Pincus, M.D.
Sandy Ferris

The Practice of Electroconvulsive Therapy: Recommendations for Treatment, Training, and Privileging

A Task Force Report of the
American Psychiatric Association

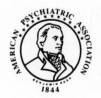

Published by the
American Psychiatric Association
1400 K Street, N.W.
Washington, DC 20005

Library of Congress Cataloging-in-Publication Data

American Psychiatric Association. Task Force on Electroconvulsive Therapy.
    The practice of electroconvulsive therapy : recommendations for treatment, training, and privileging : a task force report of the American Psychiatric Association / [the American Psychiatric Association Task Force on Electroconvulsive Therapy].
        p.   cm.
    Includes bibliographical references.
    ISBN 0-89042-229-X (alk. paper)
    1. Electroconvulsive therapy—Practice. 2. Electroconvulsive therapy. I. Title.
    [DNLM: 1. Electroconvulsive Therapy.   WM 412 A512p]
    RC485.A43 1990
    616.89′122—dc20
    DNLM/DLC
    for Library of Congress   90-239
                                                                   CIP

Contents

Cross-Reference for Recommendations and Rationale Sections

Acknowledgments

THIS TASK FORCE REPORT is the product of considerable time and effort spent not only by the members of the APA Task Force on Electroconvulsive Therapy, but also by a large number of others who graciously provided their assistance. The comments and suggestions made by individuals and groups listed in Appendix A were very much appreciated (as were those of any others who were inadvertently left off the list). The financial support and encouragement by The Division of Clinical Research, National Institute of Mental Health Contract 88M02977570ID (Robert Prien, Ph.D., Project Officer) was of particular help. Constructive advice and guidance was provided throughout by the APA Committee on Research in Psychiatric Treatments and the APA Council on Research, to which this task force reported. The staff of the APA Office of Research helped out in ways too numerous to mention. In particular, the consistent efforts of Harold Alan Pincus, M.D., Director of the Office of Research, and Sandy Ferris, Staff Assistant, are acknowledged, as are those of our primary legal consultant, Joseph Onek, Esq., of the firm Onek, Klein & Farr. Finally, the preparation of this document, and the numerous preliminary drafts which preceded the present final form, took many hours of careful, at times tedious, work on the part of a number of secretarial staff, both in the task force chairman's office, and in the offices of individual task force members and at the APA. Their efforts are greatly appreciated as well.

1

Introduction

T HE PRESENT GUIDELINES provide a basic set of recommendations to assist practitioners and facilities in the safe and effective use of electroconvulsive therapy (ECT). To this end we have attempted to make their scope as comprehensive as possible, including a discussion of the important issues of education, training, and privileging.

Following the Recommendations section is a Rationale section that provides applicable background information, including discussion of underlying issues and listing of pertinent literature citations. A Bibliography and Appendices provide additional source material of potential use to practitioners.

Over the passage of more than a half-century, the practice of ECT has evolved into a highly complex procedure about which much has been learned, but also about which many questions remain. In attempting to provide a comprehensive set of recommendations, it was necessary to include material based upon empirical data and clinical consensus in those situations where well-controlled clinical trials were either unavailable or not applicable. It was also apparent that in many cases reasonable alternative courses of action to those presented in these recommendations exist (attempts were made to cover such alternatives within the Rationale section). For these reasons, it must be understood that the recommendations provided in these guidelines represent suggestions rather than requirements.

In writing a set of recommendations covering a complex procedure such as ECT, it is impossible to cover all cases or deal with all possible exceptions. Accordingly, there will be times when a reasonable and prudent practitioner will, because of overriding factors, be justified in altering practice from that recommended herein. In addition, new information of clinical relevance is continually appearing and should be readily incorporated into clinical practice whenever clearly shown to either maximize efficacy or minimize adverse effects.

To aid the practitioner in weighing the importance of individual recommendations, we have endeavored to distinguish recommendations that we believe to be crucial to the delivery of safe and effective treatment from those that we believe to be of lesser importance. This distinction, when present, is made by the use of the categorical term "should" to cover the former case, while more equivocal terms such as "encouraged," "suggested," "recommended," or "considered" are used in the latter situation.

As a final caveat, the practitioner should be aware that legal regulations exist regarding ECT, particularly concerning informed consent procedures (see Section 5), and that these regulations vary considerably among jurisdictions. Given the widespread and time-varying nature of such regulations, it cannot be assumed that recommendations contained herein will always be compatible with requirements contained within present and future statutes. Accordingly, it is incumbent upon practitioners to seek out information on applicable regulations prior to beginning practice of ECT and to be aware of substantive statutory changes as they unfold.

The process by which these guidelines were developed has its roots in the efforts of earlier task forces and committees, both in the United States and elsewhere, which have labored over the past 50 years to help standardize and optimize the clinical practice of ECT (e.g., Group for the Advancement of Psychiatry 1947, 1950; Royal College of Psychiatrists 1977, 1989; American Psychiatric Association Task Force on ECT 1978; Pankratz 1980; Ontario Ministry of Health 1985; Consensus Conference 1985).

In particular, the 1978 APA Task Force report on ECT made many pertinent and carefully thought out recommendations regarding clinical practice. Unfortunately, many of these recommendations, especially those dealing with education and training, were not followed. In 1980 the Royal College of Psychiatrists commissioned a survey of the practice of ECT in Great Britain which found, after observing the administration of ECT in most facilities offering this treatment, that deficiencies in clinical practice were common (Pippard and Ellam 1981; Anonymous 1981). A more recent survey covering the Republic of Ireland produced similar findings (Latey and Fahey 1985).

In 1985 the National Institute of Mental Health (NIMH) and the National Institutes of Health (NIH) convened a Consensus Development Conference to consider the role of ECT in contemporary psychiatric practice (Consensus Conference 1985). While finding that ECT does indeed represent a safe and effective treatment in many cases, the panel also expressed concern that in order "to prevent misapplication and abuse, it is essential that appropriate mechanisms be established to ensure proper standards and monitoring of ECT."

In June 1987, acting upon suggestions by its membership, the APA constituted a new Task Force on Electroconvulsive Therapy to develop guidelines for clinical practice of this treatment modality. The specific charge to the task force mandated coverage of indications, contraindications, consent, technique, education, and training. The task force was also asked to provide the basis for its recommendations and to provide suggestions for how these guidelines might be implemented. The task force has received partial financial support from the NIMH (Contract 88M029775570ID), which viewed this project as consistent with the recommendations of the 1985 Consensus Development Conference on ECT.

To ensure that its product would be scientifically, ethically, and legally sound, and would be conveyed in a manner useful to clinicians, the task force sought input from a large number of professional organizations (covering the fields of psychiatry, anesthesiology, nursing, nurse anesthesia, and psychology), individual experts in related areas (including psychiatry, neurology, psychology, anesthesiology, cardiology, obstetrics, medical ethics, and law), regulatory bodies (Joint Commission on Accreditation of Healthcare Organizations [JCAHO] and the Food and Drug Administration [FDA]), and lay mental health organizations (see the list in Appendix A). To a substantial degree, the input from these diverse sources served to mold these guidelines into their present form.

We encourage ECT practitioners and trainees in related disciplines to read these guidelines and to consider their implementation. To assist in their dissemination, publication of the entire guidelines document will be supplemented by summaries of its contents in other written sources, as well as by presentations at relevant meetings and symposia. Finally, these guidelines should be viewed as part of an ongoing process of improving clinical practice, and efforts should be undertaken to update this work in the future.

2

Recommendations for Clinical Practice, Education and Training, and Privileging in Electroconvulsive Therapy

1. Introduction

1.1. Purpose and Applicability of Recommendations

These recommendations for clinical practice, education and training, and privileging seek to encourage the delivery of effective and safe electroconvulsive therapy (ECT). They should be viewed as suggestions and not as requirements. In some cases, recommendations necessarily have been based upon clinical experience, rather than rigorous data. Even when such data exist, viable alternative approaches may be present, which, under some circumstances, might be preferred. Furthermore, whenever innovations in technique become supported by newly available information, their incorporation into clinical practice should be encouraged. As with all medical care, the treating physician must take that course of action which, on the basis of data available at the time, is most compatible with safe and effective clinical management, and, where applicable, is consistent with statutes and precedents set by state and federal law.

Since these recommendations are meant to apply to a wide spectrum of clinical situations and practice settings, care has been taken to distinguish recommendations that are believed to be crucial to the delivery of safe and effective treatment from those which are felt to represent "optimum" practice. In the former case, recommendations are qualified by categorical terms such as "should," while in the latter situation, descriptions such as "encouraged," "suggested," "recommended," or "considered" are applied.

Discussion of these recommendations, as well as literature citations, are provided in the Rationale section of these guidelines.

1.2. Definitions

a) *Attending Physician:* The physician responsible for the overall treatment of the condition for which ECT is recommended.

b) *Treating Psychiatrist:* The physician(s) administering ECT (see Sections 7.2.2(a) and 16.2).

c) *Anesthetist:* The individual(s) responsible for administering anesthesia for ECT (see Sections 7.2.2(b) and 16.1).

d) *Consentor:* The individual providing informed consent for ECT (See Sections 5.2 and 5.5).

e) *Facility:* The organization responsible for the development and implementation of policies and procedures for both clinical practice of ECT and privileging of individuals in its administration (see Sections 7.1, 8.1, 11, 14, and 16).

f) *ECT Course:* A series of ECT treatments administered to induce a clinical remission in a defined episode of a mental disorder (see Sections 2, 5.2, 5.3, and 11.10.2).

g) *Continuation/Maintenance ECT:* The use of ECT to maintain an induced clinical remission and/or minimize likelihood of relapse. The onset of a period of continuation or maintenance ECT is defined as the point at which therapeutic intent shifts from inducing a remission to maintaining it (see Sections 5.2, 5.3, and 13).

2. Indications for Use

2.1. General Statement

Referrals for ECT are based upon a combination of factors, including the patient's diagnosis, nature and severity of symptomatology, treatment history, consideration of anticipated risks and benefits of viable treatment options, and patient preference. At present there are no diagnoses which should automatically lead to treatment with ECT. In most cases ECT is used following treatment failure on psychotropic agents (see Section 2.2.2), although specific criteria do exist for use of ECT as a first-line treatment (see Section 2.2.1).

2.2. When Should a Referral for ECT Be Made?

2.2.1. Primary Use of ECT

Situations where ECT may be used prior to a trial of psychotropic agents include, but are not necessarily limited to, the following:

a) where a need for rapid, definitive response exists on either medical or psychiatric grounds; or

b) when the risks of other treatments outweigh the risks of ECT; or

c) when a history of poor drug response and/or good ECT response exists for previous episodes of the illness; or

d) patient preference.

2.2.2. Secondary Use of ECT

In other situations, a trial of an alternative therapy should be considered prior to referral for ECT. Subsequent referral for ECT should be based on at least one of the following:

a) treatment failure (taking into account issues such as choice of agent, dosage, and duration of trial);

b) adverse effects which are unavoidable and which are deemed less likely and/or less severe with ECT;

c) deterioration of the patient's condition such that criterion 2.2.1(a) is met.

2.3. Major Diagnostic Indications

Diagnoses for which either compelling data are present for efficacy of ECT, or a strong consensus exists in the field supporting such use.

2.3.1. Major Depression

a) ECT is an effective treatment for all subtypes of unipolar major depression, including major depression, single episode (296.2x) and major depression, recurrent (296.3x) (American Psychiatric Association 1987).

b) ECT is an effective treatment for all subtypes of bipolar major depression, including bipolar disorder, depressed (296.5x); bipolar disorder, mixed (296.6x); and bipolar disorder, not otherwise specified (296.70).

2.3.2. Mania

ECT is an effective treatment for all subtypes of mania, including bipolar disorder, mania (296.4x); bipolar disorder, mixed (296.6x); and bipolar disorder, not otherwise specified (296.70).

2.3.3. Schizophrenia and Other Functional Psychoses

a) ECT is an effective treatment for psychotic schizophrenic exacerbations in the following situations:

   1) catatonia (295.2x); or
   2) when affective symptomatology is prominent; or
   3) when there is a history of a favorable response to ECT.

b) ECT is effective in related psychotic disorders, notably schizophreniform disorder (295.40) and schizoaffective disorder (295.70). ECT may also be useful in patients with atypical psychosis (298.90) when the clinical features are similar to those of other major diagnostic indications.

2.4. Other Diagnostic Indications

Diagnoses for which efficacy data for ECT are only suggestive, or where only a partial consensus exists in the field supporting its use. In such cases, ECT should be recommended only after standard treatment alternatives have been considered as a primary intervention. The existence of such indications, however, should not deter the use of ECT for treatment of a concurrent major diagnostic indication (Section 2.2).

2.4.1. Mental Disorders

Although ECT has sometimes been of assistance in the management of mental disorders other than those described above (Major Diagnostic Indications, Section 2.3), such usage is not adequately substantiated and should be carefully justified in the clinical record on a case-by-case basis.

2.4.2. Organic Mental Syndromes

ECT may be effective in the management of severe organic affective and psychotic conditions displaying symptomatology similar to functional diagnoses, or in treating deliria of various etiologies, including toxic and metabolic.

2.4.3. Medical Disorders

a) The neurobiologic effects associated with induced generalized seizure activity may be of benefit in treating a small number of medical disorders.

b) Such conditions include, but are not limited to:
1) catatonia secondary to medical conditions
2) hypopituitarism
3) intractable seizure disorder
4) neuroleptic malignant syndrome
5) Parkinson's disease (particularly with the "on-off" phenomenon).

3. Contraindications and Situations of High Risk

3.1. Contraindications

There are no "absolute" contraindications to ECT.

3.2. Situations Associated with Substantial Risk

a) Situations exist in which ECT is associated with an appreciable likelihood of serious morbidity or mortality. In such cases, the decision for ECT should be based upon the premise that the patient's condition is too grave, i.e., "life-threatening," to leave untreated, and that ECT is the safest treatment available.

b) In these instances, careful medical evaluation of risk factors should be carried out prior to ECT, with specific attention to treatment modifications which may diminish the level of risk (see Section 6.4).

c) Specific conditions associated with substantially increased risk include the following:
1) space-occupying cerebral lesion, or other conditions with increased intracranial pressure.
2) recent myocardial infarction with unstable cardiac function.
3) recent intracerebral hemorrhage.
4) bleeding, or otherwise unstable, vascular aneurysm or malformation.
5) retinal detachment.
6) pheochromocytoma.
7) anesthetic risk rated at ASA level 4 or 5.

4. Adverse Effects

4.1. General

a) Physicians administering ECT should be aware of the principal adverse effects which may accompany its use.

b) The nature, likelihood, and persistence of adverse effects should be considered on a case-by-case basis in the decision to recommend ECT and in obtaining informed consent (see Section 5).

c) Efforts should be made to minimize adverse effects by appropriate modifications in ECT technique and the use of adjunctive medications (see also Section 6.4).

4.2. Cognitive Dysfunction

a) Orientation and memory function should be assessed prior to ECT and periodically throughout the ECT course to detect and monitor the presence of ECT-related cognitive dysfunction (see Section 12.2.1 for details). This assessment should attend to patient self-reports of memory difficulty.

b) If a patient develops severe cognitive side effects, the physician administering ECT should review the case and take appropriate action. The contributions of medications, ECT technique, and spacing of treatments should be reviewed. Potential treatment modifications include a change from bilateral to unilateral right electrode placement, decreasing the intensity of electrical stimulation, increasing the time interval between treatments, and/or altering the dosage of medications, or, if necessary, terminating the treatment course.

4.3. Cardiovascular Dysfunction

a) The electrocardiogram (ECG) and vital signs (blood pressure, pulse, and respiration) should be monitored during each ECT treatment in order to detect cardiac arrythmias and hypertension (see Section 11.7).

b) Each facility should be prepared to manage the cardiovascular complications known to be associated with ECT. Personnel, supplies, and equipment necessary to perform such a task should be readily available (see Sections 7 and 8).

4.4. Prolonged Apnea

Resources for maintaining an airway for an extended period, including intubation, should be available in the treatment room (see Sections 7 and 8).

4.5. Prolonged Seizures

Each facility should have policies to abort prolonged seizures (see Section 11.8.4).

4.6. Treatment Emergent Mania

Rare occurrences where patients switch from depressive or affectively mixed states into hypomania or mania during a course of ECT should be distinguished from organic euphoria. Treatment strategies include continuation of ECT, delay of ECT and observation of the patient, and termination of the ECT course followed by pharmacotherapy.

4.7. Adverse Subjective Reactions

Apprehension and/or fear of ECT by patients or their families should be addressed both during the informed consent procedure (Section 5), and throughout the ECT course. The discussion of such concerns with the attending physician and/or members of the ECT treatment team is encouraged, and, where indicated, treatment procedures should be modified to alleviate such problems.

4.8. Other Adverse Effects

Headache, nausea, and muscle ache or soreness during the first few hours following seizure induction are common. Such occurrences warrant symptomatic treatment. When such effects are recurrent or particularly bothersome, prophylaxis should be considered.

5. Consent for ECT

5.1. Overview

Policies and procedures should be developed to assure proper informed consent, including when, how, and from whom it is to be obtained, and the nature and scope of information to be provided. These policies and procedures should be consistent with state and local regulatory requirements, which vary considerably by jurisdiction.

5.2. The Requirement for Consent

a) Informed consent should be obtained from the patient except in situations where the capacity to consent is lacking (see Section 5.5.3).

b) Informed consent for ECT is given for a specified treatment course or for a period of continuation/maintenance ECT (see Section 13.3), and may be withdrawn at any time, including between ECT treatments, by the individual providing consent.

5.3. When and by Whom Should Consent Be Obtained?

a) Informed consent for ECT, including the signing of a formal consent document, should be obtained prior to onset of an ECT treatment course or a period of continuation or maintenance ECT.

b) Informed consent should be obtained by the patient's attending physician, treating psychiatrist or designee, unless otherwise specified by law. When separate informed consent for ECT anesthesia is required, it should be obtained by the anesthetist or designee, unless otherwise specified by law.

c) Informed consent for ECT is a dynamic process which is not completed with the signing of the formal consent document, but continues throughout the ECT course. The consentor should be informed of substantial alterations in the treatment procedure (including a perceived need for an unusually large number of treatments—see Section 11.10.2), and any other factors having a major effect upon risk-benefit considerations. Reminding the consentor, in an ongoing fashion, that he or she may withdraw consent for ECT at any time is encouraged. Significant discussions with the consentor regarding these issues should be documented in the clinical record.

d) In the case of continuation/maintenance ECT (see Section 13.3), renewed informed consent should be obtained at least every six months.

5.4. Information to Be Conveyed

5.4.1. General Considerations

a) Information describing ECT (see below) should be conveyed by a written consent document. This document and/or a summary of general information related to ECT should be given to the consentor to keep (examples are provided in Appendix B). The use of a separate consent document for anesthesia with ECT is not generally desirable, though it may be required in certain settings.

b) The written consent document should be supplemented by an overview of general information on ECT and case-specific data presented orally by the attending physician, treating psychiatrist, or designee. The use of additional supplementary information in written, audio, or video format is encouraged.

c) All information should be provided in a form understandable to the consentor, and should be sufficient to allow a reasonable person to understand the risks and benefits of ECT and to evaluate the available treatment options.

d) The consentor should have an opportunity to ask questions relevant to ECT or to treatment alternatives.

5.4.2. Information Provided

The consent document should provide:

a) a description of ECT procedures including:
  1) when, where, and by whom the treatments will be administered
  2) a range of the number of treatment sessions likely
  3) a brief overview of the ECT technique itself.

b) a statement of why ECT is being recommended and by whom, including a consideration of reasonable treatment alternatives.

c) a statement that, as with any treatment modality, the therapeutic (or prophylactic) benefits associated with ECT may be transient.

d) a statement as to the likelihood and severity of risks related to anesthesia, muscular relaxation, and seizure induction: including mortality, cardiac dysfunction, confusion, acute and persistent memory impairment, musculoskeletal and dental injuries, headaches, and muscle pain.

e) an acknowledgment that, as with any other procedure involving general anesthesia, consent for ECT also implies consent to perform appropriate emergency medical interventions in the unlikely event that this proves necessary during the time the patient is not fully conscious.

f) an acknowledgement that consent is voluntary and can be revoked at any time before or during the treatment course.

g) a statement that the consentor is encouraged to ask questions at any time regarding ECT, and whom to contact for such questions.

h) a description of any restrictions on patient behavior which are likely to be necessary prior to, during, or following ECT.

5.5. Capacity and Voluntariness to Provide Consent

5.5.1. General Considerations

a) Capacity to provide consent for ECT is operationally defined as being able:

> 1) to comprehend the nature and seriousness of the illness for which treatment is being offered,
>
> 2) to understand the information provided concerning this treatment modality, and
>
> 3) to form a rational response based upon this information.

b) Patients are considered to have the capacity to consent for ECT unless the evidence to the contrary is compelling. The presence of psychosis, irrational thinking, or involuntary hospitalization do not in themselves constitute proof of lack of capacity. The status of patients who have previously been adjudicated legally incompetent for medical purposes may vary depending upon jurisdiction, although consent is generally provided in such cases by a legally appointed guardian or conservator.

c) Unless otherwise specified by statute, the determination of capacity to consent should be made by the patient's attending physician or designee.

d) In the event of refusal to provide or withdrawal of consent for ECT, the attending physician and/or treating psychiatrist should inform the consentor of anticipated effects of this action upon clinical course and treatment planning.

5.5.2. Patients Having the Capacity to Provide Consent

In this case, ECT should only be administered in the presence of voluntary patient agreement, including signing of a formal consent document.

5.5.3. Patients Lacking the Capacity to Provide Consent

State and local law covering consent to treatment for patients lacking the capacity to provide such consent should be followed, including statutes pertinent to emergency situations where a delay in treatment may lead to death or serious impairment in health. Applicable legal requirements vary considerably by jurisdiction and are subject to revision over time. Unless otherwise specified by law, surrogate decision makers should be provided with the information described above. When allowable, consideration should be given to any positions previously expressed by the patient when in a state of determined or presumed capacity, as well as to the opinions of major significant others.

6. Use of ECT in Special Populations

6.1. Children and Adolescents

a) The use of ECT in children and adolescents should be limited to the diagnostic indications described in Section 2.

b) Because the use of ECT in children is rare, data regarding efficacy and adverse cognitive effects in this age group continue to be sparse. Given this uncertainty, ECT in children age 12 or under should be reserved for instances where other viable treatments have not been effective or cannot be safely administered. At the same time, however, age should not be considered an absolute contraindication for the use of ECT.

c) Prior to referral for ECT, concurrence with the recommendation for ECT should be provided by two psychiatrists who are not otherwise involved with the case and who are experienced in the treatment of children. The consultants should deliver their opinion only after interviewing the patient, reviewing the clinical record, and discussing the case with the patient's attending physician.

d) The anesthetist for ECT should be experienced in anesthetic procedures with children of this age.

e) Since more experience with the use of ECT exists in the case of adolescents, and, in addition, potential risks of adverse cognitive effects are less uncertain, the procedures for referral to ECT for adolescents aged 13–17 should be as in (c) and (d) above, except that documented concurrence need be provided by a single psychiatrist with experience treating adolescents.

f) Each facility offering ECT for children and/or adolescents should develop policies covering consent to ECT for this patient population. These policies should be compatible with applicable state and federal regulations, particularly with regard to specification of circumstances under which such persons should be considered adults for purposes of consent for medical procedures (see Section 5).

6.2. The Elderly

a) ECT may be used with the elderly, regardless of age. Efficacy does not diminish with advancing age. While all somatic treatments, including ECT, are associated with increased risk in the elderly, particularly those with concurrent physical illness, clinical experience suggests that ECT may be generally less risky than pharmacotherapy in this group.

b) Dosages of anticholinergic, anesthetic, and relaxant agents may need modification on the basis of physiologic changes associated with aging.

c) The stimulus intensity should be selected with the awareness that seizure threshold generally increases with age.

d) Decisions regarding ECT technique should be guided by the possibility that ECT-induced cognitive dysfunction may be greater with the elderly.

6.3. Pregnancy

a) ECT may be used in all three trimesters of pregnancy. Although teratogenic risks of anesthetic agents during the period of embryogenesis (up to 8 weeks gestational age) are unlikely to be greater than those of psychopharmacologic alternatives, such risks should be noted in the informed consent process.

b) Obstetric consultation should be obtained prior to ECT.

c) Noninvasive monitoring of fetal heart rate during each ECT treatment session and recovery period is encouraged when gestational age is over 10 weeks.

d) Additional monitoring and the presence of an obstetrician at the time of ECT may be indicated in high risk cases or when the pregnancy is close to term.

e) Facilities administering ECT in pregnant women should assure that ready access to means of managing fetal emergencies is present.

6.4. Concurrent Medical Illness

a) The anticipated effects of the patient's medical status, including current medications, upon the risks and benefits of ECT should play a part in the decision as to whether to administer ECT.

b) The evaluation of medical conditions and their interaction with ECT should incorporate pertinent laboratory tests and specialist consultation when indicated.

c) Modifications in the ECT procedure should be utilized as a means to lower morbidity and/or augment efficacy. Such modifications may include changes in ECT technique, the use of pharmacologic agents, administration of ECT in a different hospital or clinic location, and the presence of additional medical personnel or monitoring procedures.

7. Staffing

7.1. Responsibility of Facility

a) All persons involved in the delivery of ECT should be privileged in the performance of clinical ECT-related duties by the organized medical staff of the facility under whose auspices ECT will be administered (see Section 16), or be otherwise authorized under law to carry out such duties. In the event that no such organized medical staff exists, e.g., solo or small group practice, the individual should be privileged in the ECT-related duties by another facility having an organized medical staff.

b) The director of each such facility, or his or her designee, should appoint an individual to be responsible for maintaining up-to-date policies and procedures regarding ECT, for assuring that these policies and procedures are met, and for seeing that appropriate staffing, equipment, and supplies are available.

c) Each such facility should implement a quality assurance program to monitor adherence to policies and procedures, to detect occurrences of major adverse effects, and to correct observed deficiencies.

7.2. The ECT Treatment Team

7.2.1. Members
The ECT treatment team consists of at least a treating psychiatrist, an anesthetist, and a recovery nurse. In addition, the use of an ECT treatment nurse or assistant is strongly encouraged.

7.2.2. Responsibilities
a) *Treating Psychiatrist.* The treating psychiatrist should maintain overall responsibility for the proper administration of ECT treatment. He or she should confirm that the pre-ECT evaluation has been satisfactorily completed (Section 9), and assure that the delivery of ECT is compatible with established policies and procedures (Section 11).

b) *Anesthetist.* Each facility should determine whether and under what circumstances individuals from specific disciplines, e.g., anesthesiology, nurse anesthesia, psychiatry, etc., may serve as anesthetist for ECT (see Section 16). The anesthetist should be responsible for the maintenance of an airway and oxygenation; and, with the assistance of the treating psychiatrist, the delivery of anesthetic, relaxant, and adjunctive agents and the management of emergent adverse reactions. The anesthetist should have current certification in advanced cardiac life support (ACLS) or its equivalent, and should be capable of managing foreseeable medical emergencies until other appropriate personnel are available.

c) *ECT Treatment Nurse or Assistant.* This individual should be responsible for selected tasks delegated by the treating psychiatrist and/or anesthetist. Such tasks may include education of patients and their families regarding ECT, assisting in the informed consent process, logistical coordination of treatments, readying the treatment area for administration of ECT, assistance of patients to and from the treatment area, application of stimulus and monitoring electrodes, placement of bite-block, monitoring of vital signs, documentation of treatment-related data, and assuring that ECT-related supplies, including those necessary for handling medical emergencies, are kept in stock and that relevant equipment is properly maintained.

d) *Recovery Nurse.* This person should be responsible for monitoring vital signs and mental status during the acute postictal/postanesthetic period. The recovery nurse should also be capable of monitoring and adjusting the flow of intravenous fluids, administering oxygen per mask, suctioning oropharyngeal secretions, behaviorally managing postictal disorientation and agitation, and determining when intervention by the anesthetist or treating psychiatrist is indicated. It is preferable that more than one recovery nurse be available if multiple patients will be present simultaneously in the recovery area.

8. Location, Equipment, and Supplies

8.1. Treatment Suite

The treatment suite should consist of a well lit and well ventilated treatment area, and adjoining but separate recovery and waiting areas. If feasible, the waiting area should be sufficiently separate from the treatment and recovery areas as to insulate the waiting patient from auditory and visual contact with the treatment and recovery areas, as well as from patients being transported between the latter two locations. Dedicated space should be made available within the treatment suite for ECT-related equipment, supplies, and records.

8.2. Equipment

8.2.1. Treatment Area

Equipment should be available to induce a seizure, monitor physiologic response, maintain an airway, deliver positive pressure ventilation, and provide resuscitation in case of cardiovascular or respiratory difficulties.

a) At a minimum, the following equipment should be present in the treatment area:
1) ECT treatment device (accessibility to a backup unit is encouraged)
2) device for monitoring the electrocardiogram (ECG)
3) manual sphygmomanometer or automatic device for monitoring blood pressure
4) sphygmomanometer for use in monitoring convulsion duration (Section 11.7.2.2)
5) stethoscope
6) oxygen delivery system capable of providing intermittent positive pressure oxygen by mask or endotracheal tube
7) intubation set
8) suction apparatus
9) reflex hammer
10) stretcher or bed with firm mattress and side rails, and capable of easily elevating both head and feet.

b) a defibrillator should be readily accessible for use as necessary.

c) equipment for ictal EEG monitoring is strongly encouraged (Section 11.7.2.3).

d) availability of the following additional equipment is encouraged:
1) peripheral nerve stimulator
2) pulse oximeter

8.2.2. Recovery Area

The recovery area should contain equipment to deliver intermittent positive pressure oxygen, monitor vital signs, and provide suction.

8.3. Supplies

The treatment area should have supplies to induce anesthesia, monitor physiologic function (including seizure activity), and provide ventilation and resuscitation. Suggested supplies are listed below.

8.3.1. Primary Medications (for intravenous administration unless stated otherwise)

a) primary anesthetic agent (see Section 11.3.2)
b) succinylcholine
c) anticholinergic agent(s) (see Section 11.3.1)
d) intravenous fluids (glucose in water, glucose in saline)
e) diazepam and/or alternative agents for terminating prolonged or spontaneous seizures and ameliorating postictal delirium
f) beta and alpha adrenergic blocking agents
g) nitroglycerin tablets and/or ointment
h) emergency cardiac agents sufficient for first-line management of arrhythmias, cardiac arrest, and both hyper- and hypotension
i) agents to allow initial management of anaphylactic shock
j) antinausea agents
k) physostigmine

8.3.2. Suggested Additional Medications

a) alternative anesthetic agents, e.g., pentothal, ketamine, etomidate
b) alternative/supplementary relaxant agents, e.g., atracurium or curare
c) caffeine sodium benzoate

8.3.3. Other Necessary Supplies (sufficient in amount to handle all anticipated needs)

a) masks for delivery of oxygen
b) airways (assorted sizes)
c) mouthguards (bite-blocks)—soft rubber, autoclavable
d) infusion sets
e) syringes and needles (assorted)
f) monitoring electrode pads and leads
g) electrode gel or paste
h) recording paper for monitoring use
i) alcohol, acetone, and/or ethyl acetate
j) gauze pads, tape (assorted)
k) stimulus/monitoring cables for ECT device

9. Pre-ECT Evaluation

The components of a pre-ECT evaluation should be locally stipulated. Additional tests, procedures, and consultations may be indicated, on an individual basis, e.g., per Section 6 (see Section

13.3.4 regarding continuation/maintenance ECT). Such a policy should include all of the following:

a) psychiatric history and examination to determine the indication for ECT (Section 2). The history should include an assessment of the effects of any prior ECT.

b) a medical evaluation to define risk factors (including medical history, physical examination, vital signs, hematocrit and/or hemoglobin, serum electrolytes, and electrocardiogram).

c) anesthetic evaluation, addressing the nature and extent of anesthetic risk and advising of the need for modification in ongoing medications and/or anesthetic technique.

d) informed consent (see Section 5).

e) an evaluation by an individual privileged to administer ECT (treating psychiatrist—Section 7.2.2.(a)), documented in the clinical record by a note summarizing indications and risks and suggesting any additional evaluative procedures, alterations in ongoing medications, or modifications in ECT technique that may be indicated.

10. Use of Psychotropic and Medical Agents During ECT Course

a) All ongoing psychotropic and medical agents should be reviewed as part of the pre-ECT evaluation.

b) Agents that increase morbidity or decrease the efficacy of ECT should be discontinued or decreased prior to ECT as risk-benefit considerations allow. Such drugs include benzodiazepines and most other sedative hypnotics, anticonvulsants, lidocaine and its analogs, reserpine, lithium, and theophylline. Drug half-life and withdrawal effects should be considered when discontinuing these agents.

c) In general, it is advisable to discontinue psychotropic agents prior to ECT, although this action should not prevent the institution of treatments on a timely basis. The coadministration of low to moderate dosages of neuroleptics with ECT, however, may sometimes be helpful, particularly early in the treatment course for patients with psychoses. Present evidence suggests that an appreciable drug-free period is not necessary prior to ECT for patients who have been receiving monoamine oxidase inhibitors.

d) Attention should be given to specifying which medications are to be administered prior to ECT on the day of each treatment.

11. Treatment Procedures

Local policies and procedures for the administration of ECT should be developed, as noted in Section 7.1.(b). Implementation of these policies and procedures is the responsibility of the ECT treatment team. Compliance should be monitored by an ongoing quality assurance program.

11.1. Preparation of the Patient

11.1.1. Prior to First Treatment
The treating psychiatrist should examine the medical record to assure that the pre-ECT evaluation is complete, including informed consent. A standardized summary sheet for such information may be useful.

11.1.2. Prior to Each Treatment (Responsibility of Nursing Staff)
The patient should have nothing by mouth for at least six hours prior to a treatment, except for necessary medications which may be given with a small sip of water. Observation should be employed as needed to assure that nothing is taken by mouth. The patient should be asked to void and his or her head should be checked for pins and jewelry and to assure that hair is clean and dry. Eyeglasses, contact lenses, hearing aids, and dentures should be removed, unless otherwise indicated. Gum and other foreign bodies should be removed from the mouth. Vital signs should be recorded. A standardized checklist/reporting form for documenting compliance with these procedures may be useful.

11.1.3. Prior to Each Treatment (Responsibility of Treatment Team)
Prior to anesthesia, the treating psychiatrist should check that treatment orders have been recorded and followed, and both treating psychiatrist and anesthetist should review the medical record since the last ECT treatment. A member of the treatment team should check the patient's mouth for presence of foreign bodies and loose or sharp teeth. The presence of significant problems and their management should be noted in the clinical record.

11.1.4. Intravenous Access
An intravenous access should be established and maintained until the patient is ready to leave the treatment area.

11.2. Airway Management

Airway management should be the responsibility of the anesthetist. On each treatment day prior to the first treatment the anesthetist or designee should ascertain that relevant equipment (e.g., oxygen delivery system, suctioning system, and intubation set) is functional and that necessary supplies for resuscitation are available.

11.2.1. Establishment of an Airway
The ability to adequately ventilate the patient should be assured prior to administration of the muscle relaxant agent. Intubation should be avoided unless specifically indicated.

11.2.2. Oxygenation
a) Oxygenation should be maintained using positive pressure ventilation from onset of anesthesia induction until resumption of adequate spontaneous respiration, except during application of the stimulus. Up to several minutes of preanesthetic oxygenation may be useful for patients with myocardial ischemia.

b) A concentration of 100% O_2 at a flow rate of at least 5 liters per minute and a respiratory rate of 15–20 per minute using positive pressure is suggested.

c) Supplementary oxygen should be available in the recovery area.

11.2.3. Protection of Teeth and Other Oral Structures
a) A flexible protective device ("bite-block") should be inserted prior to stimulation to protect the teeth and other oral structures. At times, additional materials may be indicated, e.g., the use of dentures to protect fragile remaining teeth.

b) The patient's chin should be held during the passage of the stimulus current to keep the jaw tight against the bite-block.

11.3. Medications Used with ECT

11.3.1. Anticholinergic
a) Muscarinic anticholinergic premedications such as atropine and glycopyrrolate are used by most practitioners to minimize the risk of vagally mediated bradyrhythmias or asystole. At present, however, there is a lack of evidence as to whether such agents should be given routinely. Anticholinergic agents are specifically indicated for patients receiving sympathetic blocking agents, or where it is medically important to prevent occurrence of a vagal bradycardia.

The practitioner should take into account muscarinic properties of any other pharmacologic agents which have been given.

b) When used, the anticholinergic premedication should be administered iv 2–3 minutes prior to anesthesia or, alternatively, im or sc 30–60 minutes prior to anesthesia induction.

c) Typical dosages for atropine are 0.3–0.6 mg administered im or sc, or 0.4–1.0 mg administered iv, and for glycopyrrolate are 0.2–0.4 mg administered im, sc, or iv.

11.3.2. Anesthetic

a) ECT should be carried out using ultra-brief, light general anesthesia.

b) The anesthetic technique for ECT differs from surgical anesthesia by the presence of generalized seizure activity, a subsequent postictal state and its concomitant physiologic effects, and the ultra-brief duration of the procedure. If anesthesia is too light, loss of consciousness may not be complete and/or autonomic arousal may occur. If anesthesia is too deep, the seizure threshold may be elevated, and treatment efficacy may be compromised.

c) Most U.S. practitioners now use methohexital, typically at a dose of 0.75–1.0 mg/kg, given iv as a single bolus. Thiopental, etomidate, or ketamine are typical alternative anesthetic agents. Regardless of agent, doses are adjusted at successive treatments to provide the desired effect.

11.3.3. Relaxant

a) Skeletal muscle relaxants should be used to minimize convulsive motor activity and to improve airway management.

b) Relaxants should be administered either following anesthesia induction or soon after injection of the anesthetic agent (rapid sequence induction). The anesthetist should assure that the patient is unconscious prior to respiratory paralysis, and that a patent airway is present.

c) Succinylcholine, 0.5–1.0 mg/kg, is the preferred relaxant agent at present in the United States, and should be given either as a single iv bolus or by drip. Patients requiring complete relaxation may need higher doses. Doses should be adjusted at successive treatment sessions to achieve the desired effect. Atracurium and curare are alternative agents.

d) The adequacy of skeletal muscle relaxation should be ascertained prior to stimulation. This can be assessed by the diminution or disappearance of knee, ankle, or withdrawal reflexes; loss of muscle tone; or failure to respond to electrical stimulation delivered by a peripheral nerve stimulator. With a depolarizing muscle blocking agent such as succinylcholine, it is unlikely that maximal relaxation has been achieved until after muscle fasciculations have disappeared.

e) A screening assay for pseudocholinesterase levels or determination of the dibucaine number should be reserved for cases where the likelihood of enzyme deficiency is significantly elevated. In patients at increased risk for prolonged apnea with standard procedures, relaxation during ECT can be achieved by either very low doses of succinylcholine or the use of alternative agents, such as atracurium.

11.4. ECT Devices

11.4.1. Device Characteristics

a) Devices used to deliver the electrical stimulus for ECT should conform to applicable national device standards.

b) Devices should allow both bilateral and unilateral stimulus electrode placement (see Section 11.5).

c) A constant-current brief pulse stimulus is recommended for routine use. There have been reports that higher energy waveforms, such as the sinewave, may be effective in otherwise refractory cases, though present evidence for such an effect is not convincing.

d) Stimulus intensity controls should allow sufficient flexibility in at least one parameter to treat patients with both low and high seizure thresholds. The device user manual should contain suggestions as to choice of stimulus parameters and dosing strategy (see Section 11.6).

e) Devices should allow control over the flow of the electrical stimulus, including the ability to abort the stimulus instantaneously.

f) The passage of the electrical stimulus should be accompanied by an auditory and/or visual indicator.

g) A means of assuring that stimulus cables are properly connected to the ECT device and that contact with the scalp is adequate is encouraged. Methods of accomplishing this task include a pretreatment "self-test" feature to measure load impedance, and an automatic stimulus abort feature that is triggered by either excessively high or low load impedance.

11.4.2. Device Testing

a) Prior to first use of a new device, output characteristics and operation of all controls, parameters, and features of the device should be tested and calibrated by qualified personnel. Test results should be documented and deficiencies corrected before subsequent use.

b) Device manufacturers should provide a description of testing procedures and suggested preventative maintenance instructions. Retesting and/or removal of the device for servicing should be carried out in cases of suspected device malfunction. The nature of deficiencies and corrective actions taken should be documented. Devices known to be malfunctioning should not be used until repaired.

c) Electrical safety testing procedures should be performed and documented prior to first use and at intervals prescribed by pertinent standards and/or local requirements regarding medical devices involving patient contact. Worn cables and connectors should be replaced.

11.4.3. Electrical Safety Considerations

a) The device's electrical grounding should not be bypassed. ECT devices should be connected to the same electrical supply circuit as all other electrical devices in contact with the patient, including monitoring equipment (see Section 11.7).

b) Grounding of the patient through the bed or other devices should be avoided, except where required for physiological monitoring (see Section 11.7).

11.5. Stimulus Electrode Placement

11.5.1. Characteristics of Stimulus Electrodes

Stimulus electrode properties should be in conformance with any applicable national device standards.

11.5.2. Maintenance of Adequate Electrode Contact

a) Adequate contact between stimulus electrodes and the scalp should be assured. Scalp areas in contact with stimulus electrodes should be cleansed and gently abraded.

b) The contact area of the stimulus electrodes should be coated with a conducting gel, paste, or solution prior to each use.

c) When stimulus electrodes are placed over an area covered by hair, a conducting medium, such as a saline solution, should be applied; alternatively, the underlying hair may be clipped. Hair beneath the electrodes should be parted prior to application of the stimulus electrodes.

d) Stimulus electrodes should be applied with sufficient pressure to assure good contact during stimulus delivery.

e) Conducting gel or solution should be confined to the area under the stimulus electrodes, and should not spread across the hair or scalp between stimulus electrodes.

f) A means of assuring the electrical continuity of the stimulus path is encouraged (see Section 11.4.1.(g)).

11.5.3. Anatomic Location of Stimulus Electrodes

a) Treating psychiatrists should be familiar with the use of both unilateral and bilateral stimulus electrode placement.

b) The choice of unilateral versus bilateral technique should be made on the basis of an ongoing analysis of applicable risks and benefits. This decision should be made by the treating psychiatrist in consultation with the consentor and the attending physician. Unilateral ECT (at least when involving the right hemisphere) is associated with significantly less verbal memory impairment than is bilateral ECT, but some data suggest that unilateral ECT may not always be as effective. Unilateral ECT is most strongly indicated in cases where it is particularly important to minimize the severity of ECT-related cognitive impairment. On the other hand, some practitioners prefer bilateral ECT in cases where a high degree of urgency is present and/or for patients who have not responded to unilateral ECT.

c) With bilateral ECT, electrodes should be placed on both sides of the head, with the midpoint of each electrode approximately one inch above the midpoint of a line extending from the tragus of the ear to the external canthus of the eye.

d) Unilateral ECT should be applied over a single cerebral hemisphere. Most practitioners using unilateral electrode placement routinely place both electrodes over the right hemisphere, since it is usually nondominant with respect to language even for the majority of left-handed individuals. Stimulus electrodes should be placed far enough apart so that the amount of current shunted across the scalp is minimized. A typical configuration involves one electrode in the standard frontotemporal position used with bilateral ECT, and the midpoint of the second electrode one inch ipsilateral to the vertex of the scalp (d'Elia placement).

e) Care should be taken to avoid stimulating over or adjacent to a skull defect.

11.6. Stimulus Dosing

a) The primary consideration with stimulus dosing is to produce an adequate ictal response (see Sections 11.8.1 and 11.8.2). Regardless of the specific dosing paradigm used, whenever seizure monitoring (see Section 11.7.2) indicates that an adequate ictal response has not occurred, restimulation should be carried out at a higher stimulus intensity. While the specific determination of when to restimulate is covered in Sections 11.8.1 and 11.8.2, the present Section addresses the choice of stimulus dosage levels themselves.

b) The choice of stimulus dosing strategy by the treating psychiatrist should consider that seizure threshold varies among patients over a 40-fold range, and generally increases over the treatment course as well. Stimuli marginally above seizure threshold may be less therapeutic than those delivered at a higher intensity, especially with unilateral electrode placement. On the other hand, grossly suprathreshold stimuli may be associated with greater cognitive side effects. Because of these issues, a "moderately" suprathreshold dosing strategy is recommended, individualized to take into account effects of sex, age, electrode placement, anesthesia dosage, and concomitant medications on seizure threshold. This dosing strategy should involve the use of either predetermined initial stimulus levels or an empirical estimation of seizure threshold.

11.7. Physiological Monitoring

11.7.1. Safety Considerations

External physiological monitoring devices connected to the patient during the passage of stimulus current should be electrically isolated. Biomedical electronics personnel should be consulted prior to the use of monitoring devices when there is uncertainty as to the presence of electrical isolation.

11.7.2. Seizure Monitoring

11.7.2.1. General Considerations

Seizure duration should be monitored to assure an adequate ictal response (see Sections 11.8.1 and 11.8.2), to detect prolonged seizure activity (Section 11.8.4), and to enable appropriate decisions to be made regarding stimulus dosing strategy (see Section 11.6). Seizure monitoring generally consists of observation of the duration of ictal motor activity (see Section 11.7.2.2) and ictal EEG activity (see Section 11.7.2.3).

11.7.2.2. Ictal Motor Activity

a) The simplest means of monitoring seizure duration is by timing the duration of convulsive movements. This measurement should be facilitated by preventing the flow of relaxant to the distal portion of an extremity (i.e., hand or foot) by inflating a blood pressure cuff, prior to relaxant infusion, substantially above the anticipated systolic pressure during the seizure.

b) If unilateral stimulus electrode placement is used, the occluded limb should be ipsilateral to the stimulated cerebral hemisphere to assure contralateral spread of the seizure activity.

c) Because ictal movements may persist for a longer time in body regions other than the cuffed extremity, the longest duration of any seizure-related motor activity should be used.

d) The duration of cuff inflation should be minimized to avoid trauma to blood vessels. Similarly, care should be taken when using this technique in cases where extreme skeletomuscular fragility is present, e.g., severe osteoporosis.

11.7.2.3. Ictal EEG Activity

a) Since scalp electroencephalographic (EEG) activity provides a more accurate representation of seizure duration than does the convulsive motor response, it is recommended that ictal EEG monitoring be carried out, on at least a one-channel basis. Monitoring of the motor response by itself may be associated with gross underestimation of true seizure duration, leading to unnecessary restimulation in some situations, and failure to detect prolonged seizures in other cases.

b) Because the ictal EEG is sometimes difficult to interpret, particularly on the basis of a single recording channel, its use should be supplemented by the "cuff" technique described in 11.7.2.2.(a).

c) EEG recording electrodes should be sufficiently far apart and in good contact with the scalp. The location of EEG monitoring leads should be based upon maximizing the detectability of ictal EEG activity.

d) EEG may be monitored either on a visual (i.e., chart recorder or video monitor) or an auditory basis.

e) The treating psychiatrist should be aware of the different manifestations of EEG seizure onset and termination as well as artifacts likely to occur during monitoring, e.g., ECG, pulse, myographic activity, and anesthesia effects.

11.7.3. Other Physiological Monitoring

11.7.3.1. Electrocardiogram

a) ECG monitoring should be carried out, on at least a single channel basis, from prior to anesthesia induction until resumption of spontaneous respiration.

b) The capacity to provide paper copy of ECG activity is encouraged.

c) If ECG paper copy recorded at a non-standard ECG recording speed is to be entered into the clinical record, the actual chart speed or labelled timing marks should be included.

11.7.3.2. Cardiovascular Vital Signs

Systolic and diastolic blood pressure, as well as heart rate or pulse, should be measured prior to anesthesia induction and at specified times or intervals throughout the procedure, including during the patient's stay in the recovery area (see Section 11.9). Such monitoring should continue until stabilization of any ECT-related changes occurs.

11.7.3.3. Oximetry

Oximetry use with ECT should be consistent with the local standard of practice for brief anesthetic procedures. Oximetry may be particularly useful in certain high risk medical cases.

11.8. Management of Missed, Abortive, and Prolonged Seizures

11.8.1. Missed Seizures

a) In the absence of seizure activity, the patient should be restimulated at a higher intensity (e.g., 25%–100% increase). In general, up to a total of four stimulations, if necessary, may be administered within a single treatment session. Each restimulation should be preceded by a 20–40 second delay to take into account the possibility of delayed seizure onset.

b) The muscular contraction that usually accompanies the delivery of the electrical stimulus should not be mistaken for a seizure.

c) Although additional doses of anesthetic or relaxant agents are not generally required in such cases, these drugs may occasionally need to be readministered.

d) Premature termination of the stimulus, poor electrode contact, disconnection of the stimulus cable, and device malfunction may each result in missed or abortive seizures. Some devices provide information as to such events, but, in any event, the electrical continuity of stimulus cables and electrodes should be checked prior to restimulation.

11.8.2. Abortive, or "Inadequate," Seizures

a) Each facility should specify the characteristics of what will be considered an abortive, or inadequate, seizure. This determination should be based at least in part upon seizure duration (e.g., less than 20–30 seconds), although available data in this regard are limited and adequate therapeutic improvement may well occur despite seizures of short duration. The modality of seizure monitoring used in this determination, e.g., motor activity or EEG, should be specified.

b) Inadequate seizures should be followed by restimulation at a higher intensity, as described in Section 11.8.1.(a) above, except that, because of the presence of a relative refractory period, a longer time interval (e.g., 60–90 seconds) should be used than in the case of a missed seizure. This prolonged waiting period increases the likelihood that additional doses of anesthetic or relaxant agents will be necessary.

11.8.3. Situations Where Increases in Stimulus Dosage Are Insufficient to Elicit an Adequate Seizure

The following techniques, alone or in combination, should be considered as means of prolonging or otherwise augmenting seizures (no specific order of importance is implied):

a) Diminish dose of anesthetic agent.

b) Diminish or omit doses of any concomitant medications with anticonvulsant action, especially benzodiazepines.

c) Provide vigorous hyperventilation prior to and during the induced seizure.

d) Ensure adequate patient hydration.

e) Use pharmacologic enhancement of seizure duration, e.g., caffeine sodium benzoate (500–2,000 mg) administered iv over a 1-minute period 2–3 minutes prior to anesthesia induction (equivalent to 250–1,000 mg of pure caffeine).

f) Use an alternative anesthetic agent with less effect upon seizure threshold and/or duration, e.g., ketamine or etomidate.

11.8.4. Prolonged Seizures

a) Seizures persisting for more than 180 seconds by motor and/or EEG criteria should be considered "prolonged." The presence of prolonged seizures may only be apparent with EEG monitoring. (However, the practitioner must be convinced in such situations that seizure activity rather than artifact is present.)

b) Prolonged seizures should be terminated pharmacologically. Initial efforts should consist of administration of an anesthetic dose of the agent used for induction of anesthesia (except with ketamine). This procedure may be repeated after 2–3 minutes if needed. If unsuccessful, a fast-acting intravenous benzodiazepine or comparable agent should be used.

c) Oxygenation should be maintained during and immediately following prolonged seizures. Intubation should be performed in cases of respiratory compromise. Cardiovascular monitoring should be continued throughout to detect the presence of adverse cardiovascular changes.

d) Repeat doses of relaxant agents should be given if convulsive motor activity persists or recurs.

e) Appropriate medical consultation should be considered if difficulties are experienced in terminating a prolonged seizure, if spontaneous seizures occur, or if neurologic or other medical sequelae appear to be present. In such cases, ECT should be resumed only after any treatable conditions known to increase the likelihood of prolonged seizures have been corrected and an assessment of applicable risk/benefit considerations has been made.

f) A decrease in stimulus intensity at subsequent treatments should be considered following a prolonged seizure, unless such a dosage had previously elicited an inadequate response.

11.9. Postictal Recovery Period

11.9.1. Management in the Treatment Area
a) The patient should not be released from the treatment area until:

1) spontaneous respirations have resumed, with adequate tidal volumes and return of pharyngeal reflexes; and
2) vital signs are sufficiently stable that the patient can return to a lower level of observation; and
3) no adverse effects requiring immediate medical evaluation or intervention are present.

b) Physiologic monitoring should continue as specified in Section 11.7.

11.9.2. Management in the Recovery Area
a) Management of the patient while in the recovery area should be under the supervision of the anesthetist or a comparably qualified individual. This individual should be readily accessible, though not necessarily present, during this time period.

b) Patients leaving the treatment area should be brought by stretcher or bed to the recovery area (see Section 8).

c) The recovery nurse(s) should provide continuous observation and supportive care (including reorientation), measure vital signs on at least 15-minute intervals beginning with the patient's arrival in the recovery area, and alert the individual providing supervision in a timely fashion of any situation potentially requiring medical intervention.

d) The patient should not leave the recovery area until he or she is awake with stable vital signs and is otherwise prepared to return to ward care or to the care of responsible significant others (if outpatient).

e) Postictal delirium and agitation should be managed either supportively or by the iv use of the anesthetic drug or a benzodiazepine sedative/hypnotic agent. When recurrent, postictal delirium can often be prevented by the prophylactic use of the above agents. In such cases, the administration of these drugs should be delayed until after return of spontaneous respiration.

11.10. Frequency and Number of Treatments

11.10.1. Frequency of Treatments

a) Usually two or three treatments per week (on nonconsecutive days) are administered. Most facilities in the United States presently use three treatments per week.

b) Some practitioners believe that transient use of daily treatments, regardless of electrode placement, may be useful early in the treatment course when a rapid onset of response is important, as in severe mania, catatonia, high suicidal risk, or severe inanition. Prolonged use of daily treatments, e.g., "regressive ECT" is associated with increased cognitive dysfunction and should be avoided.

c) A reduction in treatment frequency should be considered if delirium or severe cognitive dysfunction occurs.

11.10.2. Number of Treatments

a) The total number of ECT treatments administered should be a function of the patient's response and the severity of adverse effects. Each facility should develop a policy regarding the number of treatments after which a formal assessment of the need for continued ECT should be discussed with the consentor, as outlined in Section 5.3.(c). An ECT course generally consists of 6–12 treatments, although a plateau in response may occur either earlier or later than this. Larger numbers of treatments are more likely to be required when a change in ECT technique has taken place due to lack of response, and possibly also in some cases of schizophrenia.

b) For ECT responders, the treatment course should be ended as soon as it is clear that a maximum response has been reached. Response should be determined by changes in target symptoms (see Section 12.1), with assessment made between each ECT treatment.

c) In the absence of any discernible clinical improvement after 6–10 treatments, the indication for continued ECT should be reassessed. Consideration may be given at such times to modification of ECT technique, e.g., a change from unilateral to bilateral electrode placement, an increase in stimulus dosage levels, or the use of drugs to potentiate the ictal response.

d) Repeated courses of ECT are sometimes necessary. The decision to readminister a course of ECT within six months should take into account the presence, severity, and persistence of cognitive deficits associated with prior ECT, since cumulative effects may occur, particularly with bilateral electrode placement.

11.11. Multiple Monitored ECT

a) Multiple monitored ECT (MMECT) is defined as the delivery of more than one adequate seizure per treatment session. Advocates of this technique report that a smaller number of treatment sessions appear to be necessary to induce a therapeutic remission, although a larger number of individual seizures may be required. Since the relative benefits and risks of MMECT compared to standard ECT have yet to be adequately defined, the majority of ECT practitioners either do not use this technique or reserve its use to providing two treatments per session in cases where there is either a high anesthetic risk or an urgent need for rapid onset of therapeutic response.

b) Facilities providing MMECT should specify their procedures, which should include: the use of EEG and ECG monitoring, recommended intervals both between seizures within a treatment session and between treatment sessions, recommended and maximum number of adequate seizures to be induced per treatment session, and the manner in which anesthesia and muscular relaxation is to be handled. Information describing known differences in benefits or risks between MMECT and standard ECT should be provided to the consentor in cases where this modality is to be used.

11.12. Outpatient ECT

11.12.1. General Statement

An ECT course may be administered on an outpatient basis for a carefully selected population of patients in a facility which is properly equipped to do so. (Facilities providing outpatient ECT should monitor adherence to relevant policies and procedures.)

11.12.2. Criteria for Selection of Patients for Outpatient ECT

a) The same indications, contraindications, consent requirements, and pre-ECT evaluations as described elsewhere in these recommendations apply.

b) The nature and seriousness of the patient's mental illness at the time of ECT does not present a contraindication to management on an outpatient basis.

c) Anticipated risks associated with the ECT course are detectable and manageable either during the ECT session itself or on an outpatient basis.

d) The patient is willing and able, either individually or with the assistance of specified significant others, to comply with the behavioral limitations that are expected over this time interval (see Section 11.12.3).

e) An attending physician has been designated who will maintain overall responsibility for the case during the period over which ECT treatments are to be administered. This individual, who may be the treating psychiatrist, should be available to the patient, pertinent significant others, and the ECT treatment team as needed.

f) The ability of the patient to meet these selection criteria should be reevaluated on an ongoing basis.

11.12.3. Limitations in Patient's Behavior

The patient should follow the behavioral limitations described below. Prior to beginning outpatient ECT, each patient and, when indicated, significant other should be instructed as to the nature and duration of these limitations. The use of a written instruction sheet is encouraged. Compliance with behavioral limitations should be assessed on an ongoing basis, and patients should be reinstructed as necessary.

a) Avoid activities that are likely to be substantially impaired by anticipated adverse cognitive effects of ECT, particularly on the day of each treatment. Because such cognitive effects vary greatly as a function of ECT technique as well as on the basis of individual differences, limitations in activities should be tailored to each individual case and adjusted as indicated. In this regard, adverse cognitive effects associated with the relatively long inter-treatment intervals typically present with continuation or maintenance ECT may not persist past the day of treatment.

b) Report any adverse effects of ECT and/or apparent changes in medical condition to the attending physician and/or ECT treatment team prior to any successive treatment.

c) Follow prescribed dietary, bowel, bladder, and grooming instructions prior to each ECT treatment.

d) Abide by specified medication regime, including any medication adjustments to be made on the day of each treatment.

11.12.4. Responsibilities of ECT Treatment Team at the Time of Each Treatment

a) Prior to ECT, check compliance with instructions dealing with oral intake, voiding, cleanliness and dryness of hair, and removal of dentures and foreign bodies from the mouth. The treatment team should also assess the presence of adverse effects from earlier ECT treatments, as well as changes in the status of ongoing medical conditions whose nature may affect risks or benefits associated with ECT.

b) Space should be provided in an adjacent area for holding and observation of patients after release from the recovery area (Section 11.9.2) prior to release from the facility. Observation should be provided either by the facility's nursing staff or by the patient's family or friends.

c) It is preferred that outpatient ECT patients leave the facility after each treatment in the care of family or friends. Unless a responsible accompanying person is available, the patient should not be released until after a member of the treatment team or designee has determined that the patient's cognitive and psychomotor status is compatible with a safe journey home without assistance.

12. Evaluation of Outcome

12.1. Therapeutic Response

a) Each treatment plan should indicate specific criteria for remission.

b) Clinical assessments should be performed by the attending physician or designee and documented prior to ECT and after every 1–2 ECT treatments, preferably on the day following the treatment.

12.2. Adverse Effects

12.2.1. Cognitive Changes

a) The presence and severity of confusion and memory impairment, in terms of both objective findings and self-report, should be monitored during a course of ECT (see Section 4.2). This evaluation should include either bedside assessment of orientation and memory (both retention of newly learned material and remote recall), and/or formal test measures.

b) Assessment should be carried out prior to ECT and at least weekly throughout an ECT course. Cognitive assessment should be performed when possible at least 24 hours following an ECT treatment.

c) In the event of a substantial deterioration of orientation and/or memory function during an ECT course, modifications of the ECT procedure should be considered (see Section 4.2.(b)), and, if these effects remain present following completion of the ECT course, a plan should be made for post-ECT follow-up assessment.

12.2.2. Other Adverse Effects

Any sudden onset of new risk factors, or worsening of those present pre-ECT, should be evaluated prior to giving the next ECT treatment (see also Sections 4.3–4.6). Patient complaints concerning ECT should be considered adverse effects, in this regard.

13. Management of Patient's Post-ECT Course

13.1. General Considerations

a) Continuation therapy, typically consisting of psychotropic medication or ECT, is indicated for most patients following completion of the ECT course. Such therapy is said to begin when the therapeutic intent shifts from active treatment to prevention of relapse. Decisions not to recommend continuation therapy should be documented.

b) Continuation therapy should begin as soon as possible after termination of the ECT course, although the presence of adverse ECT effects, e.g., delirium, may necessitate a delay.

c) Unless countervened by adverse effects, continuation therapy should be maintained for at least 6 months. Patients with a high risk of recurrence and/or residual symptomatology will often require longer-term maintenance therapy.

d) The aim of maintenance therapy is to prevent recurrence of new episodes of the index disorder. It is typically defined as treatment continuing longer than 6 months following completion of the most recent ECT course. Maintenance therapy is indicated when therapeutic response has been incomplete, when a recurrence of clinical symptoms or signs has occurred, or where a history of early relapse is present.

13.2. Continuation/Maintenance Pharmacotherapy

The choice of agent should be determined by the nature of the underlying illness, a consideration of adverse effects, and response history.

13.3. Continuation/Maintenance ECT

13.3.1. Criteria for Patient Selection for Continuation ECT

a) history of recurring episodic illness which has been responsive to ECT; and

b) either 1) pharmacotherapy alone has not proven effective in preventing early relapse or cannot be safely administered for such a purpose; or 2) patient preference; and

c) the patient is agreeable to receive continuation ECT, and is capable, with the assistance of significant others when necessary, of complying with the treatment plan.

13.3.2. Frequency and Number of Treatments

a) Various formats exist for delivering continuation ECT. The timing of treatments should be individualized for each case, and should be adjusted as necessary.

b) The duration of continuation ECT should be guided by the factors described in 13.1.(b) and 13.1.(c).

13.3.3. Maintenance ECT

Maintenance ECT is indicated when a need for maintenance treatment (Section 13.1.(d)) exists in patients already receiving continuation ECT (Section 13.3.1). Maintenance ECT treatments should be administered at the minimum frequency that is compatible with sustained remission. In general this frequency will be one treatment per 1–3 months. The continued need for maintenance ECT should be reassessed at least every three months. This assessment should include consideration of both beneficial and adverse effects.

13.3.4. Pre-ECT Evaluation for Continuation/Maintenance ECT

Each facility using continuation/maintenance ECT should devise procedures for pre-ECT evaluation in such cases. The following recommendations are suggested, with the understanding that additions to and/or increased frequency of evaluative procedures should be included whenever clinically indicated.

a) Prior to each treatment:
1) interval psychiatric evaluation (this evaluation may be done monthly if treatments are more frequent than once a month)
2) interval medical history and physical examination focussing upon specific systems at risk with ECT (this exam may be done by the anesthetist at the time of the treatment session)
b) At least every three months:
1) determination by attending physician that continuation/maintenance ECT is still indicated
2) physical examination and appropriate laboratory evaluation, including hematocrit and/or hemoglobin and serum electrolytes
c) At least every three treatments:
1) assessment of cognitive function (see Section 12.2.1)
d) At least every six months:
1) consent for ECT (see Section 5)
e) At least yearly:
1) electrocardiogram.

13.3.5. Setting

Continuation/maintenance ECT may be given on either an inpatient or outpatient basis. In the latter case, the recommendations presented in Section 11.12 apply.

13.4. Continuation/Maintenance Psychotherapy

Psychotherapy, whether on an individual, group, or family basis, may, for some patients, represent a useful component of the clinical management plan following an ECT course.

14. Documentation

It is the responsibility of the facility's medical director (or medical staff, if no such individual is defined), to assure that adequate documentation regarding ECT is carried out.

14.1. Prior to a Course or Series of ECT

The treating psychiatrist should make certain that the following documentation is included in the patient's clinical record prior to ECT:

a) reasons for ECT referral, including an assessment of anticipated benefits and risks

b) mental status, including baseline information pertinent to later determinations of therapeutic outcome, orientation, and memory function

c) signed consent document

d) a statement covering other elements of the informed consent process as described in Section 5

e) a summary of the pre-ECT evaluation

f) consultation reports as indicated (see Sections 5, 6, and 9)

g) a discussion of any planned alterations in the ECT procedure

h) a justification for outpatient setting, if applicable (see Section 11.12).

14.2. During an ECT Course or Series

14.2.1. Between ECT Treatment Sessions

Notes by the attending physician or designee should be entered at least weekly in the patient's clinical record during an ECT course and, in the case of continuation or maintenance ECT, either prior to each treatment or, if such treatments occur more frequently than one per month, at least monthly. These notes should contain an assessment of therapeutic outcome and adverse effects, as delineated in Section 12. They should also justify continuation of the ECT whenever such justification is indicated by either the number of treatments (Section 11.10) or the duration of the continuation or maintenance ECT series (Section 13.3).

14.2.2. At Time of Each ECT Treatment Session

a) For each treatment session, at least the following information should be documented in the patient's clinical record:

1) baseline vital signs;

2) medication given prior to entry into the treatment room, including dosage;

3) a note by the anesthetist concerning the patient's condition during the time he/she remains in the treatment area;

4) where applicable, a note by the treating psychiatrist or anesthetist covering any major alterations in risk factors or presence of adverse effects or complications, including actions taken and recommendations made;

5) all medication given in the treatment or recovery areas, including doses;

6) stimulus electrode placement;

7) stimulus parameter settings;

8) seizure duration (noting whether motor or EEG);

9) vital signs taken in treatment room and recovery area;

10) a note by the recovery nurse or anesthetist concerning the patient's condition by the end of his/her stay in the recovery area and the occurrence and management of any complications during that time interim.

b) The recording of duplicate information to be kept in the treatment area is encouraged, especially data regarding electrode placement, device type, stimulus parameters, and seizure duration.

14.3. Following Completion of an ECT Course

The attending physician or designee should enter into the clinical record a statement including the following information:

a) a summary of overall therapeutic outcome and adverse effects experienced as a result of the ECT.

b) a plan for post-ECT clinical management, including continuation/maintenance therapy, and any plans for follow-up of adverse effects.

15. Education and Training in ECT

15.1. General Considerations

The practice of ECT has evolved considerably since its inception over 50 years ago. A steadily growing knowledge base has brought the field of ECT to the point where the old training dictum of "see one, do one, teach one" no longer applies. Instead, the extent of knowledge and skills now required to provide safe and effective ECT is such that a more comprehensive educational and training experience is indicated. Unfortunately, in many departments training in ECT has fallen behind training in other treatment modalities. Although this type of preparation is particularly important for psychiatrists, expanded opportunities are also indicated for other members of the treatment team, including anesthesia and nursing personnel. An appreciation of the role of ECT in contemporary psychiatric practice should also be considered an important aspect of general psychiatric training in medical and nursing schools, particularly given the widespread presence of misinformation in this area. Finally, as with any other evolving and highly technical medical area, a need also exists for continuing education and training.

15.2. Medical School

a) Psychiatric instructional programs for medical students should include a didactic exposure to the role of ECT in the treatment of severe mental disorders.

b) The instructional material should provide an overview of history (including social contexts), indications and contraindications, risks, mechanisms of action, and the technique of ECT itself.

c) Didactic experience should be supplemented by the opportunity to observe ECT delivery, either directly or by using videotapes.

d) The National Board of Medical Examiners should incorporate a representative number of questions concerning ECT in the psychiatric sections of their examinations.

15.3. Psychiatric Residency Programs

15.3.1. General Issues

Department chairmen and residency training directors and committees should assess their program's training in ECT on an ongoing basis and make timely efforts to correct deficiencies. ECT training should be provided by qualified and privileged individuals (see Section 16). Departments without such personnel should use consultants and/or appropriate community practitioners. The use of videotape material may be useful but should not be a substitute for in vivo clinical experience.

15.3.2. Didactic Material to Be Covered

The following ECT topics should be covered. The provision of this material should include at least four hours of lecture and discussion. Ideally, didactic instruction should take place before or during the inpatient residency experience.

a) theory and mechanisms

b) indications and contraindications

c) patient selection and evaluation

d) consent procedures, including applicable legal ramifications

e) methods of administration, including anesthetic and relaxant agents, oxygenation and airway maintenance, stimulus electrode placement, stimulus parameters and dosing, monitoring (EEG, motor convulsion, ECG, blood pressure), management of missed and otherwise inadequate seizures, and number and frequency of treatments. Situations where major options exist, e.g., electrode placement, should be discussed.

f) instrumentation, including electrical safety considerations

g) management of adverse effects during ECT, including anticipated medical emergencies

h) evaluation of therapeutic outcome

i) clinical management of patients following completion of the ECT course

j) malpractice considerations.

15.3.3. Practical Training

15.3.3.1. General Aspects

Delivery of ECT and management of patients receiving ECT by psychiatry residents should be under the supervision of staff members who are privileged in the administration of ECT. The individual(s) or committee overseeing the practice of ECT within the department as well as the residency training committee should implement this experience. The learning aspects of such practical training should be fostered, including use of materials such as journal articles, videotapes, etc.

15.3.3.2. Specific Recommendations

a) Each resident should actively participate in at least 10 ECT treatments directly supervised by a privileged treating psychiatrist, and involving at least three separate cases.

b) Each resident should actively participate in the care of at least two patients during the ECT workup and course of treatments.

c) The use of clinical case conferences and/or regular ECT rounds is encouraged.

15.3.4. Advanced Training in ECT

Elective opportunities for advanced training in ECT for residents and fellows should be available.

15.3.5. Evaluation of Resident Performance

Evaluation should be the responsibility of the training staff, via mechanisms approved by the residency training committee.

15.3.6. Record of Education and Training in ECT

The residency training committee should maintain records of the nature, scope, and extent of specific educational and training experiences related to ECT, as well as relevant performance evaluations, for residents. Records of practical training should include quantitative information necessary for assessing compliance with recommendations made in Section 15.3.3.2.

15.4. Anesthesiology Residency Programs

15.4.1. General Issues

Instruction specifically pertaining to ECT should be incorporated into anesthesia residency programs. Because the provision of anesthesia with ECT is subject to additional considerations beyond those associated with standard anesthetic practice, appropriately qualified personnel should be utilized for such purposes. Departments of anesthesiology are also encouraged to involve individuals responsible for the education of psychiatry residents in ECT into the planning and delivery of this training experience.

15.4.2. Didactic Instruction

Material should be provided as to the aims, nature, and history of ECT, indications and contraindications, pre-ECT evaluation, nature and dosing of medications commonly utilized before, during, and immediately following the procedure, oxygenation requirements, effects of hyperventilation, physiologic monitoring, electrical safety considerations, the effects of postictal state upon recovery from anesthesia, and the nature and management of potential adverse reactions.

15.4.3. Practical Training

Supervised delivery of anesthesia to patients undergoing ECT should be provided by individuals privileged in anesthesia for ECT.

15.5. Nursing Schools

a) Nursing schools are encouraged to provide formal didactic instruction on ECT, including history, indications, contraindications, risks, the pre-ECT workup, consent procedures, and a description of technique. This instruction should specifically focus upon nursing participation in ECT treatment and postanesthetic recovery (including management of emergency situations), as well as other aspects of the role of nursing personnel in the procedure.

b) Nursing educators are encouraged to incorporate observation of ECT into their psychiatric nursing training experience, either directly or via videotaped material.

c) In the case of nurse anesthetist training programs, the material described above for anesthesiology residents should be covered (see Section 15.4).

15.6. Specialty Board Examinations

Specialty boards for psychiatry, anesthesiology, and nursing should incorporate questions concerning appropriate ECT topics in their examinations, and should consider training in ECT, as described above, to be a factor in their requirements for board eligibility.

15.7. Continuing Education Program

15.7.1. General Considerations

Opportunities should be provided for practitioners to keep up to date in their knowledge and practical expertise in ECT, and to allow those whose prior training has not been sufficient to more fully develop an adequate background in this area. Although it is anticipated that the great majority of such training opportunities will be geared toward the psychiatrist, an effort should be made to also make them relevant to other disciplines involved in the practice of ECT. Attendance at continuing education programs should be a factor in privileging (see Section 16).

15.7.2. Specific Recommendations

15.7.2.1. Courses and Short-Term Fellowship Experiences

a) Relevant professional organizations and facilities offering ECT are encouraged to develop clinically oriented continuing education programs on ECT, including provision of continuing medical education (CME) credit. When feasible, such programs should incorporate hands-on experience in addition to didactic material. The American Psychiatric Association should take a major role in this effort by the inclusion of clinically relevant material on ECT in the scientific program of its annual meeting.

b) Available courses and fellowship opportunities should be publicized (see Appendix C). In each case it should be made clear whether the course offers a comprehensive overview or whether it is oriented toward a single issue, e.g., ECT in the medically ill.

15.7.2.2. Lectures and Symposia

Both clinically and research oriented lectures and symposia focusing on ECT-related topics should be encouraged at the local, national, and international level by professional organizations, relevant academic departments, and facilities providing ECT. In addition, courses directed towards the management of disorders for which ECT may be indicated are encouraged to consider including material concerning the specific role of ECT.

15.7.2.3. Reference Materials

Medical and nursing schools as well as hospitals and clinics providing ECT are encouraged to have available a variety of reference material applicable to ECT, including videotapes, books, professional journals (especially *Convulsive Therapy*), and copies of relevant published reviews and clinical and research reports (see Appendix C).

16. Privileging in ECT

16.1. General Considerations

a) Each member of the ECT treatment team, as defined in Section 7, should be clinically privileged to practice his or her respective ECT-related duties or be otherwise authorized by law to do so. Such privileging should be carried out according to procedures established by the organized medical staff of the facility, or its equivalent, under whose auspices ECT is administered. Where applicable, the medical staff organization is encouraged to meet requirements of state, federal, and voluntary surveying bodies. In the absence of an organized medical staff, or of a specific department or service within the facility, privileging by the medical staff of a separate facility meeting these requirements should be obtained. In any case, ongoing quality assurance mechanisms should be used to monitor the privileging and clinical performance of treatment team members, with corrective action taken as indicated.

b) Recommendations for privileging in ECT for treating psychiatrists are provided below. Although recommendations for selection and privileging of other members of the ECT treatment team are beyond the scope of the present document, facilities offering ECT are encouraged to develop the means to establish that such individuals have received adequate training, such as that outlined in Section 15, and have demonstrated clinical competency in relevant areas (see Section 7).

16.2. Suggested Criteria for Privileging of Psychiatrists to Administer ECT

16.2.1. General Issues

a) It is the responsibility of the medical director of each facility under whose auspices ECT is administered to assure the clinical competency of treating psychiatrists. Privileges to administer ECT should be given only to individuals with demonstrated proficiency to deliver ECT in a safe and effective manner in keeping with established clinical practice.

b) The medical director, with the assistance of the individual or committee responsible for overseeing policies and procedures regarding ECT and other organizational components or outside consultants that are deemed relevant, should develop a formal written plan for the provision and maintenance of ECT privileges. This plan should include the designation of those responsible for determining whether criteria for privileging have been met. The proceedings of all privileging actions should be documented.

c) In the event that ECT is to be provided in a setting without a medical director, policies and procedures should be implemented regarding privileging which are compatible with those outlined otherwise in this Section. Ongoing monitoring of compliance with these policies and procedures should be undertaken via a quality assurance program or equivalent process, with corrective action taken as indicated.

16.2.2. Specific Criteria for Privileging

a) The candidate's education, training, experience, and history of privileging in ECT should be reviewed by the body designated for this purpose (see 16.2.1). The material considered should include items such as medical licensure, board certification, evidence of satisfactory completion of residency training, records of relevant residency and CME educational and training experiences (both didactic and practical), holding of malpractice insurance covering practice of ECT, and letters of recommendation specifically directed toward the candidate's education, training, experience and competency in ECT. The information provided should be sufficient to determine whether the candidate's training and experience are sufficient to meet the suggested education and training criteria delineated in Section 15.

b) If this evaluation indicates that the candidate is competent to practice ECT, then he or she may be granted clinical ECT privileges following satisfactory administration of ECT, as observed by a designated in-house evaluator, or, if necessary, by an outside consultant. Prior to delivery of the first of such treatments, the candidate should become familiar with the facility's policies and procedures for ECT, as well as the layout of the ECT treatment suite and the use of applicable ECT devices, seizure monitoring equipment, and ECT supplies.

c) Should the initial evaluation raise questions as to the proficiency of the candidate to administer ECT, he or she should be requested to undertake an appropriate training experience. This training may involve either attendance at an organized ECT course, or the use of a structured clinical practicum experience supplemented by supervised reading. In either case, supervised administration of at least 10 ECT treatments should be required. In such cases privileges may then be awarded after completion of all of the following:

1) satisfactory completion of the prescribed training experience
2) completion of the orientation process as described in Section 16.2.2.(b)
3) demonstration of proficient administration of ECT in the local setting.

16.2.3. Maintenance of Privileging

The maintenance of ECT privileges should be determined on the basis of continued proven clinical proficiency. Reassessment of privileges should be undertaken at least every two years or as may be otherwise specified by regulation or local policy for clinical privileges in general. The plan developed by the facility for this purpose should contain the following components:

a) use of the quality assurance program to monitor selected aspects of performance by the ECT treatment team. The plan should incorporate a mechanism by which any apparent deficits are subject to institutional review and are followed by corrective action.

b) ongoing monitoring of numbers of ECT administered by treating psychiatrists, so that individuals whose practice becomes inactive can be given the opportunity to demonstrate use of proficient technique upon resumption of an active clinical role.

c) demonstration of continued education in ECT-related areas.

3

Rationale for Recommendations

1. Introduction

The preceding recommendations were developed from extensive experience and a large body of literature. The present rationale clarifies and supports these recommendations, provides further information and references to the literature, and discusses areas in which diverse practice options exist. Each major section corresponds to the identically numbered section in the recommendations, and should be viewed in the context of that document. In order to maintain continuity within the rationale, some degree of redundancy between it and the recommendations was unavoidable.

2. Indications for Use

The decision to use ECT in an individual case results from a risk/benefit analysis, taking into account the severity of the illness, the treatment history, the anticipated efficacy and safety of ECT in the condition, and the likely efficacy and safety of alternative treatments. In most instances, the illness is sufficiently severe as to warrant hospitalization, and other treatments have either proven ineffective or are inapplicable for various reasons.

Like the indications for most medical treatments, today's usage of ECT is defined by controlled trials, uncontrolled clinical reports, case studies, and opinion surveys. This literature has been recently reviewed by Weiner and Coffey (1988) and by Abrams (1988).

Referral for ECT

Primary use. ECT is a major treatment in psychiatry, with well defined indications. It should not be seen only as a "last-resort" therapy; such a view may well deprive patients of effective treatment. In some situations, its action may be more rapid than that of psychotropic drugs, suggesting that where a more rapid response is required, as when patients are severely medically ill, or at risk to harm themselves or others, primary use of ECT should be considered. In other situations, ECT may represent the safest treatment alternative available. Other considerations for first-line use of ECT relate to the patient's treatment history and his/her treatment preferences. A past successful response to ECT, particularly in the context of present, or even past, drug refractoriness or intolerance, represents an indication for early consideration of ECT.

Some practitioners also base a decision for primary use of ECT upon other factors, including nature and severity of symptomatology. Severe major depression with delusions or catatonic symptoms and manic delirium are examples of circumstances for which a clear consensus exists favoring early reliance on ECT.

Secondary use. ECT is most often used in patients when other treatments have failed. Medication resistance, sensitivity to side-effects, deterioration in condition, the appearance of a suicidal drive, or inanition are reasons to refer for ECT on this basis.

The definition of medication resistance and its implications with respect to a referral for ECT have been the subjects of considerable discussion (Quitkin et al. 1984; Kroessler 1985; Keller et al. 1986; Sackeim et al., 1990). At present no accepted standards exist. In practice, psychiatrists rely upon factors such as type of agent used, dosage, treatment duration, adverse effects, patient age, nature and degree of therapeutic response, and type and severity of clinical symptomatology, in making their determinations. Patients with psychotic depression should not be viewed as nonresponders unless a trial of an antipsychotic agent has been considered, generally in combination with an antidepressant drug. Similarly, patients not responding to psychotherapy alone should not be considered treatment resistant in the context of a referral for ECT, regardless of diagnosis.

In general, failure of severely ill psychiatric patients to respond to antidepressant drug trials does not preclude a favorable response to ECT (Avery and Lubrano 1979; American Psychiatric Association 1978; Fink 1979, 1987a; Abrams 1988), although recent data suggest that refractoriness may be higher in such a population (Prudic et al., in press).

Major Diagnostic Indications

Diagnostic classification.   Much of our information concerning the efficacy of ECT predates the present diagnostic terminology which was adopted by the American Psychiatric Association in 1980 and revised in 1987 (American Psychiatric Association 1980, 1987). Many illnesses described in the new classification are reminiscent of old typologies, but others are more complex, and translations are difficult. Accordingly, it must be understood that controlled studies are not available for each diagnostic entity.

Major depression.   The efficacy of ECT in depressive mood disorders is documented in extensive studies, beginning with the clinical "open" trials of the 1940s (Kalinowsky and Hoch 1946, 1961; Sargant and Slater 1954); the comparative ECT/drug therapy trials of the 1960s; ECT versus sham-ECT trials, both in the 1950s and in the more recent British trials (Abrams 1988); and the recent comparative trials of ECT technique assessing the contributions of electrode placement and stimulus type and intensity to clinical efficacy (Malitz and Sackeim 1986; Weiner et al. 1986b).

While ECT was introduced as a treatment for the psychoses of dementia praecox, early trials quickly found it even more effective in patients with affective disorders, both in the depressive and manic phases. This literature is summarized by Kalinowsky and Hoch (1946):

> It was not until several years after the introduction of convulsive therapy that its usefulness in affective disorders was recognized. . . . Since then it has become the treatment of choice for these conditions. The responses of the various types of depressions are so similar that it is safe to assume a close relation or even the same underlying process in manic-depressive depressions, involutional depressions, senile depressions. (Kalinowsky and Hoch 1946, p. 169)

These authors also note: "The rate of remissions in manic-depressive depressions in most reports varies between 80–100%" (Kalinowsky and Hoch 1946, p. 170).

Similar conclusions are cited by the British authors Sargant and Slater (1954):

> From their use in schizophrenia, convulsions came to be tried in depressive states, and here the results were even more brilliant (than in dementia praecox) and have stood the test of time. . . . Convulsive therapy has proved our most powerful

weapon in the treatment of (depressive syndromes of later life), and figures of from 70 to 80% recoveries are constantly being reported. (Sargant and Slater 1954, p. 80)

The results of these early studies have been more recently summarized by the American Psychiatric Association (1978), Fink (1979), Abrams (1988), and Kiloh et al. (1988).

With the introduction of the tricyclic antidepressant (TCA) and the monoamine oxidase inhibitor (MAOI) medications, questions of the relative efficacy of drugs and ECT led to random assignment trials in depressed patients in which ECT was compared with either TCA or MAOI, and/or with either placebo or "sham-ECT" (involving anesthesia without the passage of the stimulus current). These studies demonstrate a superiority in antidepressant efficacy for ECT compared to sham-ECT and placebo, and equivalent or superior effects with respect to tricyclic and monoamine oxidase inhibitor antidepressant drugs. In particular, recent British studies found a significant advantage in antidepressant activity for real versus sham-ECT (Freeman et al. 1978; Johnstone et al. 1980; Lambourn and Gill 1978; West 1981; Brandon et al. 1984; Gregory et al. 1985).

In terms of investigations which specifically focussed on ECT versus antidepressant drugs, three studies which meet modern standards of random assignment and blind ratings found a significant therapeutic advantage for ECT over tricyclic antidepressants and placebo (Greenblatt et al. 1964; Medical Research Council 1965; Gangadhar et al. 1982). Other studies also report ECT to be as or more effective than TCA (Bruce et al. 1960; Kristiansen 1961; Norris and Clancy 1961; Robin and Harris 1962; Fahy et al. 1963; Stanley and Fleming 1962; Hutchinson and Smedberg 1963; Wilson et al. 1963; McDonald et al. 1966; Davidson et al. 1978) or monoamine oxidase inhibitors (Corsellis and Meyer 1954; King 1959; Kiloh et al. 1960; Stanley and Fleming 1962; Hutchinson and Smedberg 1963; Davidson et al. 1978).

Additional studies report effective antidepressant treatment by ECT in patients who have been refractory to other forms of treatment (Fink 1987a). The DeCarolis study, reviewed by Avery and Lubrano (1979), is a case in point. DeCarolis treated 437 depressed patients with 200 to 350 mg/day of imipramine. Of 109 patients who failed this therapy after 30 days, 93 (85%) responded to a course of 8–10 bilateral ECT. Similar success for ECT after drug therapy failure is reported by Kantor and Glassman (1977), Minter and Mandel (1979), Paul et al. (1981); Magni et al. (1988), and Sackeim et al. (in press).

ECT is an effective antidepressant in all subtypes of major depressive disorder. Available evidence suggests that degree of improvement seems more related to the severity of the illness rather than to presence of a specific diagnostic subtype (Hamilton 1986). Specifically, subtyping as to unipolar versus bipolar form of illness has generally not been found to be related to short-term clinical outcome (Abrams and Taylor 1974; Perris and d'Elia 1966; Black et al. 1987a; Aronson et al. 1988). Similarly, while clinical lore argues that the presence of melancholia or vegetative symptoms is predictive of good outcome with somatic antidepressant treatments, including ECT, research efforts have failed to consistently find that the presence or degree of melancholia and/or vegetative symptoms predicts ECT response (Zimmerman et al. 1985).

Still, the presence of certain symptoms may be of prognostic utility with ECT, particularly with respect to delusions (Clinical Research Centre 1984; Janicak et al. 1989). Most depressed patients with delusions fare poorly with antidepressant drugs alone (Kroessler 1985), and the use of ECT or the combination of antipsychotic and antidepressant drugs is indicated.

The presence of catatonia or catatonic symptoms is also a favorable prognostic sign. Catatonia occurs in patients with severe affective disorders (Abrams and Taylor 1976; Taylor and Abrams 1977), some severe medical illnesses (Breakey and Kala 1977; O'Toole and Dyck 1977; Hafeiz 1987), as well as among patients with schizophrenia. Regardless of diagnosis, ECT is effective in relieving the syndrome, even in its more malignant form of "lethal catatonia" (Mann et al. 1986; Geretsegger and Rochawanski 1987) (a phenomenon which may be related to neuroleptic malignant syndrome [Pearlman 1986; Kellam 1987; Addonizio and Susman 1987; Casey 1987; Weiner and Coffey 1987]).

The studies reported by Avery and Winokur (1976, 1977) and McCabe (1976) suggest that treatment with ECT is more effective than alternative treatments for severe depressive disorders, resulting in a lower incidence of suicide. The efficacy of ECT in resolving suicidal drive is reportedly limited to the index treatment, however, and long-term suicide rates seem not to be affected (Milstein et al. 1986).

Major depression which occurs in individuals with coexisting psychiatric and medical disorders is termed "secondary depression." In general, patients with secondary depression respond less well to somatic treatments than those with primary depressions (Bibb and Guze 1972; Zorumski et al. 1986; Black et al. 1987b). However, there is sufficient variability in outcome with ECT that each case of secondary depression must be considered on its own merits. In a

relative sense, patients with anxiety disorders, schizophrenia, sub-
stance abuse, borderline syndrome, hysterical personality, and hy-
pochondriacal features have been reported to respond less favorably
to ECT (Taylor 1982; Weiner and Coffey 1987). On the other hand,
patients with post-stroke depression (Murray et al. 1986; House
1987; Allman and Hawton 1987; deQuardo and Tandon 1988) or
"schizoaffective disorder" (Tsuang et al. 1979; Pope et al. 1980; Ries
et al. 1981; Black et al. 1987b) are believed to have a relatively good
prognosis with ECT. Patients with coexisting diagnoses of both
major depression and dysthymia present special problems in that
both diagnostic assessment and determination of baseline affective
status are often difficult. Still, even though dysthymia does not
respond to ECT, its presence should not deter the treatment by ECT
of a coexisting major depression, as long as it is understood that
residual dysthymic symptomatology may be present (Weiner and
Coffey 1987).

Mania. Mania is a syndrome which, when full blown, is potentially life-threatening on the basis of exhaustion, excitement, and
violence. ECT is rapidly effective in mania (Kalinowsky and Hoch
1961; McCabe 1976; McCabe and Norris 1977; Fink 1979; Small
1985). However, since the introduction of antipsychotic drugs and
lithium, ECT has only been used occasionally, primarily in therapy
resistant or intolerant cases. Retrospective analyses of the efficacy
and safety of ECT and lithium (with or without antipsychotic drugs)
find both to be roughly equivalent in efficacy (Thomas and Reddy
1982; Black et al. 1987c; Alexander et al. 1988). In recent controlled
prospective studies, ECT is found as effective or more so than
pharmacotherapy, although sample sizes are small (Milstein et al.
1987; Mukherjee et al. 1987; Small et al. 1988).

The rare syndrome of manic delirium represents a primary
indication for the use of ECT, as it is rapidly effective with a high
margin of safety (Constant 1972; Heshe and Roeder 1975; Kramp
and Bolwig 1981). In addition, manic patients who cycle rapidly may
be particularly unresponsive to medications, and in such instances
ECT may represent an effective alternative treatment (Berman and
Wolpert 1987).

Schizophrenia. ECT has been widely used for patients with
schizophrenia (American Psychiatric Association 1978; Shugar et al.
1984), although in recent years its utility has been questioned (Klein
et al. 1980). In the first decades of its use, convulsive therapy was
seen as an effective treatment for psychotic manifestations in patients with dementia praecox, particularly those whose duration of

illness was relatively brief (Meduna 1937; Kalinowsky and Hoch 1961; Sargant and Slater 1964).

At present, ECT is generally considered in drug-refractory or intolerant cases, particularly when distinct psychotic episodes are characterized by catatonic or affective symptoms or when there is a history of a positive response to ECT. Particularly in young patients, it may be difficult to determine whether the episode is a manifestation of an affective or a schizophrenic disorder. Recent controlled investigations have shown that some schizophrenic episodes respond rapidly to ECT, especially when affective symptoms are prominent (Taylor and Fleminger 1980; Brandon et al. 1985; Gregory et al. 1985). In addition, recent prospective comparisons of such patients treated with antipsychotic drugs or ECT find the two regimens equivalent (Bagadia et al. 1983; Janakiramaiah et al. 1982). Others have found good results in patients with schizoaffective or schizophreniform disorder (Tsuang et al. 1979; Pope et al. 1980; Ries et al. 1981; Black et al. 1987b). Another area of recent investigation has been the potentiation of ECT response with concurrent neuroleptic agents (Small et al. 1982; Janakiramaiah et al. 1982). Such data require further corroboration before firm conclusions can be drawn.

Chronic cases, or those without the presence of favorable symptomatologic profiles, are considerably less likely to respond to ECT (Salzman 1980; Small 1985), although comparable efficacy to that of neuroleptic agents may still be present as long as a distinct psychosis exists (May 1968). In effect, the limitation of ECT to drug-refractory cases in some clinical trials may have acted to minimize estimates of the efficacy of ECT in a more general schizophrenic population (Weiner and Coffey 1987).

Other Diagnostic Indications

ECT has been used successfully in some other conditions, although this utilization has been rare in recent years (American Psychiatric Association 1978). Much of this usage has been reported as case material, however, and typically reflects the use of ECT only after all other treatment options have been exhausted or when the patient presents with life-threatening symptomatology. Because of the absence of controlled studies, which would, in any event, be difficult to carry out given the low utilization of ECT in these situations, any such referrals for ECT should be adequately substantiated and documented in the clinical record. The use of psychiatric and/or medical consultation by individuals experienced in the management of like conditions may be a useful component of the evaluative process.

Mental disorders. Other than the major diagnostic indications discussed above, evidence for efficacy of ECT in the treatment of functional mental disorders is not compelling, although reports of favorable outcome exist for some conditions, e.g., severe obsessive compulsive disorder (Gruber 1971; Dubois 1984; Mellman and Gorman 1984; Janike et al. 1987; Khanna et al. 1988). As noted earlier, major diagnostic indications for ECT may coexist with other conditions, and practitioners should not be dissuaded by the presence of secondary diagnoses from recommending ECT when it is otherwise indicated, e.g., a major depressive episode in a patient with dysthymia.

Organic mental and medical disorders. Severe organic affective and psychotic conditions, as well as certain types of deliria, may be responsive to ECT, although its use in such situations is rare and should be reserved for patients who are refractory and/or intolerant to more standard medical treatment regimens, or who require an urgent response. Prior to ECT, attention should be given to the evaluation of the underlying etiology for such problems. Conditions where ECT has been reported to be of benefit include alcoholic delirium (Dudley and Williams 1972), toxic delirium secondary to agents such as phencyclidine (PCP) (Rosen et al. 1984; Dinwiddie et al. 1988), and in organic mental syndromes related to lupus erythematosus (Guze 1967; Allen and Pitts 1978; Douglas and Schwartz 1982; Mac and Pardo 1983) and enteric fevers (Breakey and Kala 1977; O'Toole and Dyck 1977; Hafeiz 1987).

When evaluating potential organic mental syndromes, it is important to recognize that confusional syndromes or cognitive impairment may accompany a major depressive disorder, amounting to what has been termed "pseudodementia" or "reversible dementia." Occasionally, the cognitive impairment may be sufficiently severe to mask the presence of affective symptomatology. When such patients have been treated with ECT, recovery has often been dramatic (Allen 1982; McAllister and Price 1982; Grunhaus et al. 1983; Burke et al. 1985; Bulbena and Berrios 1986; O'Shea et al. 1987; Fink 1989).

Physiologic effects associated with ECT (Lerer et al. 1986; Malitz and Sackeim 1986; Abrams 1988) may also have a direct therapeutic effect on certain medical disorders, apparently independent of antidepressant, antimanic, and antipsychotic actions. Because of the usual presence of viable treatment alternatives in such cases, ECT should be reserved for use on a secondary basis. Medical conditions which have been reported to have improved following ECT include neuroleptic malignant syndrome (Pearlman 1986; Hermle and Oepen 1986; Pope et al. 1986; Kellam 1987; Addonizio and Susman 1987; Casey 1987; Weiner and Coffey 1987; Hermesh et al. 1986), iatrogenic hypopituitarism (Pitts and Patterson 1979), and intractable epilepsy and persistent status epilepticus (Sackeim et al. 1983; Schnur et al. 1989). In terms of the latter indication, the rise in seizure threshold produced by ECT may reduce the incidence of spontaneous seizures and interrupt certain types of status epilepticus (Dubovsky 1986; Hsiao et al. 1987).

Another medical condition for which there has been considerable recent research interest with respect to ECT is Parkinson's disorder, where ECT has been shown to induce a transient reduction in the severity of muscular rigidity and improvement in motor function (Lebensohn and Jenkins 1975; Dysken et al. 1976; Ananth et al. 1979; Atre-Vaidya and Jampala 1988; Roth and Mukherjee 1988). Patients with the "on-off" phenomenon, in particular, show considerable improvement (Balldin et al. 1980, 1981; Ward et al. 1980; Andersen et al. 1987). Given the presence of substantial numbers of treatment refractory and/or intolerant patients with Parkinson's disorder, assessment of a possible role for continuation ECT should be carried out.

3. Contraindications and Situations of High Risk

In the first decades of the use of ECT, treatments were administered under a wide variety of conditions, to a wide range of patients. The principal risks were those of fear on the part of patients who were treated without anesthesia, fractures, prolonged or spontaneous seizures, amnestic or organic confusional states, cardiac or cerebral decompensation, and death. When fatalities with ECT were examined, it was observed that an appreciable minority occurred in patients with pre-existing brain lesions, and the attitude developed that a brain tumor was an absolute contraindication to ECT. Other "relative" contraindications were also described, including recent myocardial infarction, musculoskeletal disease, severe hypertension, cardiac arrhythmia, etc. As experience using ECT in patients with severe medical conditions increased, procedures were developed to minimize risks. We now understand that no contraindication to ECT is absolute, and indeed, even relative contraindications are few. Instead, it is more pertinent now to talk in terms of the level of risk rather than in terms of contraindications.

Substantial risk. Some conditions substantially increase the risk of treatment. For each decision to treat, the attending physician and treating psychiatrist must undertake a "benefit-risk" analysis of the patient's condition—the severity and duration of the illness and its threat to life; the likelihood of therapeutic success with ECT; the medical risks of ECT; and the benefits and risks of alternative treatments and of no treatment. After such an analysis, a choice can be made regarding the optimal intervention for an individual patient. In treating "high-risk" patients with ECT, attempts should be made to improve and stabilize risk-related medical conditions (see Section 6.4). Careful medical and neurological evaluations often are an essential component to this process, as may be consultations with internists, cardiologists, neurologists, and other specialists (see Section 9).

Conditions which may substantially increase the risk of treatment with ECT include space-occupying brain lesions and other causes of increased intracranial pressure, recent myocardial infarction, recent intracerebral hemorrhage, bleeding or otherwise unstable aneurysms or vascular malformations, and other conditions associated with markedly increased anesthetic risk (e.g., American Society of Anesthesiologists [ASA] level 4 or 5). The concept of "recency" as it applies to these conditions is difficult to define in the absence of relevant supporting data. In effect, absolute time periods represent only one component of such a determination, as, for example, lesions heal at different rates in different situations. Accordingly, the risks associated with a mild myocardial infarction without adverse sequelae at six weeks following the insult may be less than those present at six months following a severe, poorly compensated event.

In assessing risk levels, physicians should focus carefully on the extent to which the medical condition adversely affects body physiology, such as increased cerebrospinal fluid pressure, blood pressure, or intraocular pressure; instability of heart rate and cardiac output; or additional factors which might otherwise increase anesthetic risk. It should be understood that this process requires the presence of a well-trained, highly skilled clinical team. This evaluation should also consider whether and how the treatment procedure can be modified to ameliorate risks. Often such treatment modifications can substantially lower risks to acceptable levels, particularly when the risks associated with alternative treatment options are not inconsequential. For patients with intracranial tumors, for example, the review by Maltbie et al. (1980) and recent clinical reports of successful ECT treatment of patients with certain types of brain tumors (Fried and Mann 1988; Greenberg et al. 1988) outline potential ECT treatment modifications that can be used in such conditions.

4. Adverse Effects

Medical complications. The mortality associated with ECT is estimated to be approximately the same as that associated with general anesthesia in minor surgery. This rate is approximately one death per 10,000 patients treated (Abrams 1988). The rate of significant morbidity and mortality is believed to be lower with ECT than with administration of antidepressant medications, despite the frequent use of ECT in patients with medical complications and in the elderly (Weiner and Coffey 1987, 1988).

When mortality occurs during a course of ECT, it typically happens immediately following the seizure or during the postictal recovery period. Cardiovascular complications are the leading cause of death and of significant morbidity (Pitts 1982; Prudic et al. 1987; Welch and Drop 1989). Cerebrovascular complications are notably rare. Given the high rate of cardiac arrhythmias in the immediate postictal period, the majority of which are benign and resolve spontaneously, ECG should be monitored during and following the procedure (see Section 11) and patients should not be taken to the recovery area until there is resolution of significant arrhythmias (e.g., bigeminy). Vital signs (pulse, systolic and diastolic pressure) should be stable prior to the patient's leaving the recovery room (Section 11.9). It is believed that patients with pre-existing cardiac illness are at greater risk for post-ECT cardiac complications (Prudic et al. 1987).

Two other possible sources of morbidity are prolonged seizures and tardive seizures. Management of prolonged seizures is described in Section 11. Failure to terminate seizures within a period of 3 to 5 minutes may increase postictal confusion and amnesia. Inadequate oxygenation during prolonged seizures may increase the risk of hypoxia and cerebral dysfunction, as well as cardiovascular complications. In animal studies, seizures that are sustained continuously for periods exceeding 30 minutes, regardless of steps taken to maintain appropriate levels of blood gases, are associated with an increased risk of structural damage and cardiovascular and cardiopulmonary complications (Ingvar 1986; Siesjö et al. 1986). Prolonged seizures may be more likely in patients receiving medications that lower seizure threshold (e.g., theophylline, high dosage neuroleptics) (Devanand et al. 1988a), in patients receiving concomitant lithium therapy (Weiner et al. 1980), in patients with pre-existing electrolyte imbalance, and possibly with the repeated induction of seizures within the same treatment session (Strain and Bidder 1971).

There has been some concern as to whether the rate of spontaneous seizures is increased following the course of ECT (Assael et al. 1967; Devinsky and Duchowny 1983). The available evidence, however, indicates that such events are extremely rare and probably do not differ from population base rates (Blackwood et al. 1980; Small et al. 1981). There are no data concerning rates of tardive seizures, i.e., seizures that occur following termination of the ECT-induced seizure, but experience indicates that these are also rare events. As noted in Section 11.8, tardive seizures occurring during the immediate postictal period are not necessarily accompanied by motor manifestations, underscoring the desirability of seizure EEG monitoring.

Other medical side effects of ECT that have been reported include headache, nausea, muscle ache or soreness, weakness, drowsiness, anorexia, and amenorrhea (Sackeim et al. 1987a). Headache and nausea are frequently observed during and shortly following the postictal recovery period and typically subside with symptomatic treatment.

Medical adverse events can, to some extent, be anticipated. Whenever possible, such effects should be minimized by modifications in ECT procedures. Patients with preexisting cardiac illness, compromised pulmonary status, a history of CNS insult, or medical complications following prior courses of anesthesia or ECT are likely to be at increased risk (Weiner and Coffey 1988). Treating psychiatrists should review the medical workup and history of prospective ECT patients (see Section 9). Specialist consultations or additional laboratory studies may be called for. In spite of careful pre-ECT evaluation, medical complications may arise which have not been anticipated. ECT facilities should be staffed with personnel prepared to manage potential clinical emergencies and should be equipped accordingly (see Sections 7 and 8). Examples of these events include cardiovascular complications (such as cardiac arrest, arrhythmias, ischemia, hyper- and hypotension), prolonged apnea, and prolonged or tardive seizures.

Major adverse events that occur during or soon after the ECT course should be documented in the patient's medical record. The steps taken to manage the event, including specialist consultation, use of additional procedures, and administration of medications, should likewise be documented. As cardiovascular complications are the most likely source of significant adverse events and are seen most frequently in the immediate post-ECT period, it may be useful for facilities to have a set of written procedures determined in advance to manage major cardiovascular complications. Such procedures should be modified as needed given the circumstances of individual patients. Predetermined procedures for dealing with instances of prolonged or tardive seizures may also be helpful.

Cognitive side effects. Cognitive changes associated with ECT have been the focus of intense investigation (Squire 1986). ECT is associated with a range of cognitive side effects including, but not limited to, a period of confusion immediately following the seizure, and anterograde and retrograde memory disturbance during the treatment course (Daniel and Crovitz 1986; Sackeim et al. 1986a). The available evidence indicates that these side effects subside during the weeks following the treatment course (Weiner et al. 1986a). Patients may, however, have permanent loss of specific memories for some events that occur over the months immediately preceding, during, and following the treatment course (Squire 1986). Other than these lacunae, objective testing does not indicate that capacities to acquire new information or to remember information from the past are persistently impaired by ECT (Squire 1986; Taylor et al. 1982; Weeks et al. 1980). A small minority of patients, however, report persistent deficits (Freeman and Kendell 1986). The basis of these complaints is not well understood.

Patients vary considerably in the extent and severity of short-term cognitive side effects experienced with ECT. The factors that contribute to these individual differences have not been clearly delineated. However, it is believed that patients with pre-existing cognitive impairment, neuropathological conditions (e.g., stroke), and those receiving any of a variety of psychotropic medications during the ECT course may be at increased risk for more profound cognitive side effects.

To determine the occurrence and severity of cognitive changes during and following the ECT course, orientation and memory functions should be assessed prior to initiation of ECT and throughout the course of treatments (see Section 12 for details).

The method of ECT administration strongly impacts on the extent and severity of cognitive side effects. In general, as described in Table 1, bilateral electrode placement, sine wave stimulation, high intensity stimulation, closely spaced treatments, and high dosage of barbiturate anesthetic agents are all independently associated with more intense cognitive side effects than unilateral non-dominant

Table 1. Treatment factors that may increase or decrease the
severity of adverse cognitive side effects

Treatment factor	Associated with increased cognitive side effects	Steps to be taken to reduce cognitive side effects
Stimulus waveform	Sine wave	Change to brief pulse
Electrode placement	Bilateral	Change to right unilateral
Stimulus intensity	Grossly suprathreshold	Decrease electrical dose
Spacing of treatments	ECT administered 3–5 times per week	Decrease frequency or stop ECT
Number of seizures per session	Multiple (two or more) seizures per session	Change to conventional ECT
Concomitant psychotropic medications	Lithium, benzodiazepines, neuroleptics, antidepressants	Reduce dose or stop psychotropics
Anesthetic medications	High dose may contribute to amnesia	Reduce dose as appropriate for light level of anesthesia

electrode placement, brief pulse waveform, lower intensity stimulation, more widely spaced treatments, and lower dosage of barbiturate anesthesia (Miller et al. 1985; Sackeim et al. 1986a; Weiner et al. 1986a). Optimization of these parameters can minimize short-term cognitive side effects. In patients who develop severe cognitive side effects, such as an organic brain syndrome, the attending physician and treating psychiatrist should review and adjust the treatment technique being used, (e.g., switching to unilateral ECT, lowering the electrical dosage administered, and/or increasing the time interval between treatments) and modify dosages of any medications being administered that may exacerbate cognitive side effects.

Treatment emergent mania. As with pharmacological antidepressant treatments, a small minority of depressed patients or patients in mixed affective states switch into hypomania or mania during the ECT course (Devanand et al. 1988b). In some patients, the severity of manic symptoms may worsen with further ECT treatments. In such cases, it is important to distinguish treatment emergent manic symptoms from organic euphoria. There are a number of phenomenologic similarities between the two conditions. Still, in organic euphoria patients are typically very confused and have a pronounced memory disturbance. Confusion should be continuously present and evident from the period immediately following the treatment. In contrast, manic symptomatology may occur in the context of a clear sensorium. Evaluation of cognitive status may be particularly helpful in distinguishing between these states. Organic euphoric states are often characterized by a giddiness in mood or "carefree" disposition. Classical features of hypomania, such as racing thoughts, hypersexuality, irritability, etc. may be absent. There is no established strategy on how to manage emergent manic symptoms during the ECT course. Some practitioners continue ECT to treat both the mania and any residual depressive symptomatology. Other practitioners postpone further ECT and observe the patient's course. At times, manic symptomatology will remit spontaneously without further intervention. Should the mania persist, or the patient relapse back into depression, reinstitution of ECT may be considered. Yet other practitioners terminate the ECT course and start pharmacotherapy, often with lithium carbonate, to treat emergent manic symptomatology.

Adverse subjective reactions. Negative subjective reactions to the experience of ECT should be considered as adverse side effects. Prior to ECT, patients often report apprehension; rarely, some patients develop intense fear of the procedure during the ECT course. Family members are also frequently apprehensive about the effects of the treatment. As part of the consent process prior to the start of the ECT course, patients and family members should be given the opportunity to express their concerns and questions to the attending physician and/or members of the ECT treatment team (see Section 5). Since much of such apprehension may be based on lack of information, it is frequently helpful to provide patients and family members with an information sheet describing basic facts about ECT (see Section 5). This material should be supplemental to the consent form. It is also useful to make available video material on ECT. Addressing the concerns of patients and family members should be a process that continues throughout the course. In centers that regularly conduct ECT, it has been found useful to have ongoing group sessions, led by a member of the treatment team, for patients receiving ECT and/or their significant others. Such group sessions, including prospective and recently treated patients and their families, may engender mutual support among these individuals and can serve as a forum for education about ECT.

5. Consent for ECT

Overview

"The core notion that decisions regarding medical care . . . are to be made in a collaborative manner between patient and physician" has, over the last few decades, evolved into a formal legal doctrine of informed consent (Applebaum et al. 1987, p. 12). Unfortunately, there has been a notable absence of medical, legal, and regulatory consensus concerning the fundamental parameters that constitute informed consent for ECT, or, for that matter, other medical and surgical treatments: What is informed consent? Who should provide consent, and under what circumstances? How, and by whom, should capacity for consent be determined? What information should be provided to the consentor and by whom? And how should consent be managed with incompetent and with involuntary patients? General reviews of informed consent issues as they relate to ECT can be found in Parry (1986), Roth (1986), Taub (1987), and Winslade (1988), while capacity for consent and the use of ECT in incompetent and/or involuntary patients is specifically addressed in Roth et al. (1977), Salzman (1977), Culver et al. (1980), Roy-Byrne and Gerner (1981), Gutheil and Bursztajn (1986), Mahler et al. (1986), Applebaum et al. (1987), and Wettstein and Roth (1988).

The psychiatric profession, both in the United States and elsewhere, has made a number of attempts to offer practical guidelines for the implementation of consent in the clinical setting. In this regard, the conceptual requirements for informed consent posed by the 1978 APA Task Force on ECT, are still perceived to be applicable: 1) the provision of adequate information, 2) a patient who is capable of understanding and acting intelligently upon such information, and 3) the opportunity to provide consent in the absence of coercion (American Psychiatric Association 1978). It should be understood that specific recommendations concerning consent for ECT at times must reflect a trade-off between the preservation of the autonomy of the patient, on the one hand, and the assurance of the patient's right to receive treatment on the other.

On an individual basis, a crucial hallmark of informed consent, above and beyond compliance with specific recommendations, is the quality of ongoing interactions between the consentor and the physician. In general, the more the physician keeps the consentor abreast of what is transpiring in the case, the more he/she allows the consentor to be involved in everyday decision making, and the more he/she is sensitive to the consentor's concerns and feelings regarding these decisions, the fewer problems there will be with consent. While many patients referred for ECT do not wish and/or are not capable of taking such an active role in management decisions, it is incorrect to assume that this is always the case.

Informed consent for ECT is mandated, both on an ethical basis and by regulation, and it is incumbent upon facilities using ECT to implement and monitor compliance with reasonable and appropriate policies and procedures. Although the practitioner must, by law, be bound to applicable state and local regulatory requirements concerning consent for ECT, efforts should be made via judicial and political action to correct occurrences of overregulation (Winslade et al. 1984; Taub 1987). In this regard, ECT should not be considered different from other medical or surgical procedures with comparable anticipated risks and benefits. Regulations should not unduly stand in the way of the patient's right to treatment, since unnecessary suffering, increased physical morbidity, and even fatalities may result if procedures to provide ECT to incompetent or involuntary patients (see below) are needlessly prolonged (Mills and Avery 1978; Roy-Byrne and Gerner 1981; Tenenbaum 1983; Walter-Ryan 1985; Miller et al. 1986).

When and by Whom Should Consent Be Obtained?

As with all cases involving consent for medical and surgical procedures, the patient, i.e., the individual on whom the procedure will be carried out, should, unless lacking capacity (see below) or otherwise specified by law (see Section 6.1), be the one to provide informed consent. The involvement of significant others in this process should be encouraged (Consensus Conference 1985), but should not be required (Tenenbaum 1983).

ECT is unusual, but not unique, among medical procedures in that it involves a series of separate, though identical, interventions spaced over an appreciable time period (typically 2 to 4 weeks for an ECT course). Because it is the series of treatments, rather than any given individual treatment within the series, that is responsible for both the benefits and adverse effects associated with the procedure, consent for ECT should apply to the treatment series as a whole.

Since a considerable time period is involved, however, care should also be taken to ensure that the informed consent process continues across the complete period during which ECT is administered. Patient memories of consent for medical and surgical procedures in general are commonly faulty (Roth et al. 1982; Meisel and Roth 1983). For patients receiving ECT, this difficulty with recall may be exacerbated by both the underlying illness and the treatment itself (Sternberg and Jarvik 1976; Squire 1986). For these reasons, the consentor should be reminded in an ongoing fashion of his/her option to withdraw consent. This reminding process should also include a periodic review of clinical progress and side effects.

The occurrence of a substantial alteration in the treatment procedure or other factor having a major effect upon risk-benefit considerations should be conveyed to the consentor on a timely basis. The need for ECT treatments exceeding the range originally conveyed to the consentor as likely (see Section 11.10) represents one such example. All consent-related discussions with the consentor should be documented by a brief note in the patient's clinical record.

Continuation/maintenance ECT (see Section 13) differs from a course of ECT in that its purpose is the prevention of relapse or recurrence, and that it is characterized by both a greater inter-treatment interval and a less well-defined endpoint. Because the purpose of continuation/maintenance treatment differs from that used in the management of an acute episode, new informed consent should be obtained prior to its implementation. As a series of continuation ECT typically lasts at least 6 months, and because continuation/maintenance ECT is, by its nature, provided to individuals who are in clinical remission and who are already knowledgeable regarding this treatment modality, a 6-month interval before readministration of the formal consent document is adequate.

There is no clear consensus as to who should obtain consent. Ideally, consent should be obtained by a physician who has both an ongoing therapeutic relationship with the patient and, at the same time, has knowledge of the ECT procedure and its effects. In practice this can be accomplished by the attending physician, treating psychiatrist, or their designees acting individually or in concert.

Information Provided

The use of a formal consent document for ECT ensures the provision of at least a minimum measure of information to the consentor, although consent forms vary considerably in scope, detail, and readability. For this reason, a sample consent form and sample supplementary patient information material are included in Appendix B. If these documents are used, appropriate modifications should be made to reflect local conditions. It is also suggested that any reproductions be in large type, to ensure readability by patients with poor visual acuity.

Earlier task force recommendations (American Psychiatric Association 1978), other professional guidelines, and regulatory requirements (Mills and Avery 1978; Tenenbaum 1983; Winslade et al. 1984; Taub 1987; Winslade 1988), as well as a growing concern regarding professional liability, have encouraged the use of more comprehensive written information as part of the ECT consent process. Such material is often contained wholly within the formal consent document, while others use an additional supplementary patient information sheet. A copy of the major components of such information should be given to the consentor to facilitate learning and understanding of the material and assimilation by significant others.

To rely entirely upon the consent form as the sole informational component of the informed consent process would be ill-founded. Even with considerable attention to readability, many patients understand less than half of what is contained in a consent form (Roth et al. 1982). It is interesting to note, however, that psychiatric patients do not perform more poorly than medical or surgical cases (Meisel and Roth 1983). Besides problems with limited patient comprehension, members of the treatment team may see the consent form as relieving them of any additional responsibility to supply information to the patient/consentor over the ECT course. Alternatively, the consentor may perceive the signing of the consent form as a single, final act in the consent process, after which the matter is "closed." Both of these attitudes should be eschewed.

The written information supplied within and accompanying the consent document should be supplemented by a discussion between the consentor and the attending physician, treating psychiatrist and/or designee, that highlights the main features of the consent document, provides additional case-specific information, and allows an exchange to take place. Examples of case-specific information include: why ECT is recommended, specific applicable benefits and risks, and any planned major alterations in the pre-ECT evaluation or the ECT procedure itself. Again, as with all significant consent related interactions with the patient and/or consentor, such discussions should be briefly summarized in the patient's clinical record.

To improve the understanding of ECT by patients, consentors, and significant others, many practitioners use additional written and audiovisual materials, which have been designed to cover the topic of ECT from the layman's perspective. Videotapes, in particular, may be helpful in providing information to patients with limited comprehension, although they may not serve as a substitute for other aspects of the informed consent process (Baxter et al. 1986). A partial listing of such materials has been included as part of Appendix C.

The scope and depth of informational material provided as part of the consent document should be sufficient to allow a reasonable person to understand and evaluate the pertinent risks and benefits of ECT as compared to treatment alternatives. Since individuals vary considerably in terms of education, intelligence, and cognitive status, efforts should be made to tailor information to the consentor's ability to comprehend such data. The practitioner should be aware that too much technical detail can be as counterproductive as too little.

The specific topics to be covered in the consent document generally include the following: 1) a description of the ECT procedure; 2) why ECT is being recommended and by whom; 3) applicable treatment alternatives; 4) the likelihood and anticipated severity of major risks associated with the procedure, including mortality, adverse effects upon cardiovascular and central nervous systems, and common minor risks; 5) a description of behavioral restrictions that may be necessary during the pre-ECT evaluation period, the ECT course, and the recuperative interval; 6) an acknowledgement that consent for ECT is voluntary and can be withdrawn at any time; and 7) an offer to answer questions regarding the recommended treatment at any time, and the name of whom to contact for such questions.

The description of the ECT procedure should include the times when treatments are given (e.g., Monday, Wednesday, Friday mornings), general location of treatment (i.e., where treatments will take place), and typical range for number of treatments to be administered. In the absence of precise quantitative data, the likelihood of specific adverse effects is generally described in terms such as "extremely rare," "rare," "uncommon," and "common" (see Section 4). Because of ongoing concern regarding cognitive dysfunction with ECT, an estimate of the potential severity and persistence of such effects should be given (see Section 4). In light of the available evidence, "brain damage" need not be included as a potential risk.

Capacity and Voluntariness to Provide Consent

Informed consent is defined as voluntary. In the absence of consensus as to what constitutes "voluntary," it is defined here as the consentor's ability to reach a decision free from coercion or duress.

Since the treatment team, family members, and friends all may have opinions concerning whether or not ECT should be administered, it is reasonable that these opinions and their basis be expressed to the consentor. In practice, the line between "advocacy" and "coercion" may be difficult to establish. Consentors who are either highly ambivalent or are unwilling or unable to take full responsibility for the decision (neither of which are rare occurrences with patients referred for ECT) are particularly susceptible to undue influence. Staff members involved in clinical case management should keep these issues in mind.

Threats of involuntary hospitalization or precipitous discharge from the hospital due to ECT refusal clearly represent a violation of the informed consent process. However, consentors do have the right to be informed of the anticipated effects of their actions on the patient's clinical course and the overall treatment plan. Similarly, since physicians are not expected to follow treatment plans which they believe are ineffective and/or unsafe, an anticipated need to transfer the patient to another attending physician should be discussed in advance with the consentor.

It is important to understand the issues involved in a consentor's decision to refuse or withdraw consent. Such decisions may sometimes be based upon misinformation or may reflect unrelated matters, e.g., anger towards self or others or a need to manifest autonomy. In addition, a patient's mental disorder can itself severely limit the ability to cooperate meaningfully in the informed consent process, even in the absence of psychotic ideation.

Patients who are involuntarily hospitalized represent a special case. A number of suggestions have been offered to help guarantee the right of such individuals to accept or refuse specific components of the treatment plan, including ECT. Examples of such recommendations include the use of psychiatric consultants not otherwise involved in the case, appointed lay representatives, formal institutional review committees, and legal or judicial determination. While some degree of protection is indicated in such cases, overregulation will serve to limit the patient's right to receive treatment.

Informed consent requires a patient who is capable of understanding and acting intelligently upon information provided to him/her. For the purpose of these recommendations, the term "capacity" reflects this criterion. There is no clear consensus as to what constitutes "capacity for consent." Here, a definition is proposed that the patient 1) comprehends the nature and seriousness of his or her illness, 2) understands the information provided concerning the recommended treatment, and 3) is able to form a rational response based upon this information.

The process of determining capacity for consent is not usually specified within regulations. Unless otherwise mandated by statute, this determination should be made by the attending physician or designee. There are several reasons for this view. First, the attending physician is in an excellent position to assess the patient's ability to meet the above three criteria for capacity to consent. Next, the attending physician is likely to be aware of how the patient's mental illness affects these criteria, and, in addition, to be cognizant of the relative benefits and risks for both ECT and treatment alternatives. Furthermore, the attending physician is also in a position to be aware of the feelings of the patient's significant others with respect to ECT. Finally, the attending physician is generally the one who makes such determination with respect to other medical and surgical procedures. Should the attending physician be in doubt as to whether capacity to consent is present, use may be made of an appropriate physician consultant not otherwise associated with the case.

Criteria for capacity to consent are vague, and formal "tests" of capacity do not exist. It is suggested, instead, that the individual obtaining consent consider the following in making a determination. First, capacity for consent should be assumed to be present unless compelling evidence to the contrary exists. Second, the occurrence of psychotic ideation, irrational thought processes, or involuntary hospitalization do not in themselves constitute such evidence. Third, the patient should demonstrate sufficient comprehension and retention of information so that he/she can reasonably make a decision whether or not to consent for ECT.

There is concern that attending physicians may be biased to find that capacity for consent exists when the patient's decision agrees with their own. In this regard, however, ECT should not be considered different from other treatment modalities. Fixed requirements for a priori review of capacity to consent for ECT by consultant, special committee, appointed lawyer, or judicial hearing are impediments to the patient's right to treatment and are inappropriate.

For patients who have capacity to consent, ECT should only be administered with full patient agreement. To do otherwise would infringe upon the right to refuse treatment. Potential exceptions, e.g., patient refusal when treatment is viewed as lifesaving, may be pursued judicially or as otherwise stipulated by local regulation. Situations where the patient lacks capacity to consent for ECT are generally covered by regulations which include how and from whom surrogate consent may be obtained. Patients who agree to receive ECT but are determined to lack capacity to provide informed consent, may, if legally allowable, have surrogate consent provided by a significant other (spouse, parent, sibling, or adult child). In such instances, all the information typically provided regarding ECT and alternative treatment should be shared with the significant other.

6. Use of ECT in Special Populations

Children and adolescents. Few studies cover the use of ECT in childhood or adolescence, in part because ECT is only rarely used in such a setting, in part because affective syndromes in children and adolescents are not often recognized, and in part because of theoretical concerns that induced seizures may be more toxic in these age groups. The paucity of experience and virtual absence of controlled studies make the decision to use ECT complex, and concurrence in the diagnosis and severity of the disorder and the relative merits of ECT versus treatment alternatives is important.

The indications for the use of ECT in children and adolescents are similar to those for adults (see Section 2). The child's neurophysiological and developmental maturity must be taken into consideration. In particular, some case reports suggest that when an affective syndrome is well defined, the response to ECT may be favorable (Warneke 1975; Carr et al. 1983; Black et al. 1985; Knitter 1986; Berman and Wolpert 1987; Guttmacher and Cretella 1988). Each institution should establish policies for the use of ECT in minors, including informed consent procedures. Because of the very limited experience with ECT in children, the decision for treatment should be made following concurrence by two consultants experienced in treating mental disorders of this age group. The treatment goals should be clearly defined and documented. Because of the greater experience with ECT in adolescents, and because of a greater acceptance within the field that ECT has a distinct role in this population, one consultant should suffice.

Elderly. Advanced age is not an impediment to the use of ECT. The efficacy of ECT among elderly depressed patients is high, and case reports attest to the safe use of ECT in patients up to the age of 102 years. But ECT in the elderly also presents certain age-related issues that must be considered. With increasing age, seizure threshold may rise, and effective seizures may be difficult to induce (Sackeim et al. 1987d). Attending physicians should consider the reduction or withdrawal of sedative/hypnotic agents, especially benzodiazepines; replace prophylactic lidocaine by another anti-arrhythmic drug (Hood and Mecca 1983; Devanand and Sackeim 1988); use minimal doses of barbiturate anesthesia; ensure adequate ventilation; and augment seizures, e.g., by use of intravenous caffeine, when seizure duration is deemed inadequate (Shapira et al. 1985,1987; Coffey et al. 1987; Hinkle et al. 1987). In addition, because of altered metabolism in the elderly, dosages of all medications used with ECT may need to be reduced.

Some elderly patients may have an increased likelihood of appreciable memory deficits and confusion during the course of treatment, and individuals in this age group should be carefully assessed on an ongoing basis for such changes (see Section 12). Electrode placement, stimulus intensity, and frequency of treatments (e.g., twice instead of three times weekly) should be modified as needed to minimize such effects when present.

Pregnancy. In general, recent case material supports the use of ECT as a treatment with low risk and high efficacy in the management of appropriate disorders in all three trimesters of pregnancy (Nurnberg and Prudic 1984; Repke and Berger 1984; Dorn 1985; Oates 1986; Chang and Renshaw 1986; Wisner and Perel 1988). It should also be kept in mind that lack of effective treatment may affect the health and welfare of both the patient and the fetus.

In patients with affective episodes and/or psychoses occurring during the first trimester of pregnancy, the risks of teratogenesis in the developing fetus must be considered. Lithium and benzodiazepines carry defined risks and the morbidity associated with antipsychotic and antidepressant drugs is still unknown. Most practitioners, however, consider ECT relatively safe in this regard. Although the risk of teratogenesis resulting from barbiturate anesthesia is not well understood, brief exposures to such agents are not likely to be problematic.

When gestational age is at least 10 weeks, consideration should be given to noninvasive monitoring of fetal heart rate at each treatment, so that signs of fetal distress can be detected. Some practitioners recommend the use of intubation for advanced pregnancies, because of the increased risk of gastric reflux and subsequent aspiration. It is recommended that an obstetrician be consulted prior to ECT, to clarify the risks for both patient and fetus and to suggest any treatment modifications that may be indicated. In high risk cases, additional monitoring may be needed. Facilities intending to use ECT in pregnant women should have resources available to manage foreseeable adverse effects, including the precipitation of labor (though this has not yet been reported with ECT).

Postpartum affective states. Severe depressive or manic states, with or without psychosis, occurring after childbirth are responsive to ECT (Protheroe 1969; Herzog and Detre 1976; Robinson and Stewart 1986).

Concurrent medical illness. Implications of coexisting medical illness must be considered in the decision to use ECT. The extent to which physiologic events associated with the anesthesia and induced seizure activity affect such conditions is of particular importance. Medical illnesses should be delineated and treatment instituted prior to ECT. At times, laboratory evaluation and specialist consultations are indicated. ECT technique should be modified as needed in terms of both use of pre-medications and changes in technical aspects of the treatment, e.g., dosage of medications given at the time of the treatment, electrode placement, electrical dosage, etc. In high risk cases, or where special monitoring needs exist, the presence of medical consultants at one or more of the treatments may be helpful. When risks are extremely high, ECT may need to be administered in a setting capable of providing a higher level of acute medical or surgical intervention than would otherwise be available.

Case reports describe the successful use of ECT in many conditions, ranging from pheochromocytoma (Carr and Woods 1985; Simon and Evans 1986) to vascular anomalies (Pomeranze et al. 1968; Husum et al. 1983; Greenberg et al. 1986) to those receiving anticoagulants (Tancer et al. 1987). Description of the ECT treatment of patients with cardiovascular disorders may be found in Gerring and Shields (1982), Regestein and Reich (1985), Dec et al. (1985), Burke et al. (1985), and Rodin and Voshart (1986), while the use of ECT in patients with neurological disorders is described by Dubovsky (1986) and Hsiao et al. (1987). More general reviews by Selvin (1987), Weiner and Coffey (1987), Abrams (1988, 1989b), and Fink (1988) provide further helpful information for management of ECT patients with medical disorders.

7. Staffing

Treatment team. ECT is a complex procedure which requires the presence of a well-trained, competent staff of professionals to be administered in a safe and effective fashion. ECT is not a treatment to be delivered by unskilled trainees acting without proper supervision. All members of the treatment team should be privileged in the performance of their ECT-related duties by the organized medical staff of the facility under whose auspices ECT will be delivered (see Section 16), or be otherwise authorized by law to do so. The assurance of the quality of the ECT treatment staff is sufficiently important that practitioners operating outside the context of an organized medical staff, e.g., solo or small group practice, should be concurrently privileged for ECT-related duties by a facility meeting this criterion.

Facilities offering ECT should designate an individual or committee to oversee the development of and compliance with policies and procedures for ECT, including those related to staffing, equipment, and supplies. Furthermore, facilities should implement a quality assurance program to monitor adherence to policies and procedures and occurrences of major adverse effects. Any observed deficiencies should be corrected. The ECT treatment team functions as a unit. The team typically consists of a treating psychiatrist, an anesthetist, an ECT treatment nurse or assistant, and one or more recovery nurses. When properly qualified (see below), the treating psychiatrist may also perform the duties of the ECT treatment nurse or the anesthetist. However, because of the need for at least two health care professionals in the treatment area during the administration of ECT, the treating psychiatrist may not subsume all three of these roles simultaneously. For each position on the treatment team, the pool of available staff members should be kept small to maximize continuity of care and to ensure that each individual has sufficient ongoing experience to maintain proficiency in his/her work.

Treating psychiatrist. Because his or her training and experience regarding ECT is the most comprehensive, the treating psychiatrist should maintain the overall responsibility for the administration of ECT. The treating psychiatrist is also responsible for 1) evaluating the patient prior to ECT, 2) assuring that the pre-ECT evaluation has been satisfactorily completed and documented (see Section 9), and 3) assuring that the delivery of ECT is compatible with established policies and procedures (see Section 11).

Practice varies as to whether the treating psychiatrist oversees all other aspects of the patient's mental health care during the ECT course, or whether a separate attending physician fulfills this latter function. Ideally, the same individual functions as both treating psychiatrist and attending physician. When such functions are separate, it is necessary for both physicians to be in agreement with respect to important treatment decisions such as the ECT referral and the number and type of ECT treatments provided. However, it must be stressed that in his or her capacity of maintaining overall responsibility for ECT treatment, the treating psychiatrist must have complete authority over whether and how each treatment is administered (except for anesthetic considerations). The concept of the treating psychiatrist as a "button-pusher" is incompatible with quality care.

Anesthetist. The administration of ECT, even for a procedure as short as ECT, requires skill in airway management, use of ultra-brief anesthetic and relaxant agents, and in managing potential acute adverse effects, including administration of cardiopulmonary resuscitation. If appropriately trained and privileged to perform such duties (see Sections 15 and 16), a nurse anesthetist or the treating psychiatrist him- or herself may serve in this capacity. However, high-risk cases which require more complex anesthetic management may require the presence of a qualified anesthesiologist.

Treatment nurse. The role of the ECT treatment nurse or assistant varies somewhat from location to location. In most cases, this individual is a registered nurse whose responsibilities include assisting the treating psychiatrist and anesthetist in such duties as logistical coordination of treatments, readying the treatment area for administration of ECT, helping patients to and from the treatment area, application of stimulus and monitoring electrodes, and monitoring vital signs. Many facilities have provided a much more comprehensive role for the ECT treatment nurse or assistant, including assisting with patient and family education, informed consent procedures, and documentation and overseeing the availability and function of ECT-related equipment and supplies.

Recovery nurse. The recovery nurse, generally a registered nurse, is responsible, under the supervision of the anesthetist or comparably qualified professional, for the management of the patient while in the recovery area. Duties include monitoring vital signs, mental status, and intravenous fluids. The recovery nurse should be capable of administering oxygen and suctioning and providing supportive care for postictal disorientation and agitation. Recovery area staffing should be sufficient to ensure adequate performance of these duties at all times.

8. Location, Equipment, and Supplies

Treatment suite. The treatment suite consists of three separate areas: a waiting area, where patients are temporarily placed prior to entering the actual treatment area; a treatment area, where the treatments are administered; and a recovery area, where patients are monitored and reoriented after leaving the treatment area. Facilities providing outpatient ECT (see Section 11.12) should provide an additional area for patients and significant others to wait, both prior to the patient's entering the regular waiting area and after leaving the recovery area. The various areas should be as close as possible to each other for logistical purposes, but should also be sufficiently separated that patients in one area are visually and auditorially isolated from patients and staff in other areas. Facilities should make sure that sufficient dedicated space is available in the treatment area for ECT-related equipment and supplies.

The ideal location of the treatment suite is determined by the desired attributes, e.g., access to resources necessary to treat medical emergencies, sufficient space and lighting to carry out treatments and recovery in a safe unencumbered fashion, a comfortable and unthreatening environment for patients, and a reasonable proximity to psychiatric inpatient units. Because of the need to have ready access to equipment, supplies, and personnel necessary for emergency management, some facilities locate the treatment suite either in or adjacent to outpatient or inpatient surgical areas or intensive care units. It should be understood that, even though such arrangements may be logistically unavoidable, they are likely to be suboptimum in other ways, and ongoing efforts should be made to ensure that the environment is kept as comfortable and unthreatening for patients as possible. For this reason, the routine use of a surgical operating theater, with the attendant rules of sterility and scheduling, should be avoided.

The treatment room includes devices to induce seizures and related supplies; medical equipment and supplies for prevention and management of untoward events; a source of oxygen and means for its delivery; and monitoring instruments for blood pressure, heart rate, and ECG. Medical supplies to treat cardiac and respiratory emergencies and prolonged seizures should be available. Modern ECT instruments often include capacity for EEG monitoring, a feature which is extremely useful in determination of seizure adequacy and detection of prolonged seizures (see Sections 11.7 and 11.8). Practitioners using ECT devices without EEG monitoring should consider the addition of external EEG monitoring equipment, taking care that this use does not present electrical safety problems (see Section 11.4). The presence of a back-up ECT device is helpful, in that continuity of care can be guaranteed.

9. Pre-ECT Evaluation

Although components of the evaluation of patients for ECT will vary on a case-by-case basis, each facility should devise a minimal set of procedures to be undertaken in all cases. A psychiatric history and examination, including past response to ECT and other treatments, is important to ensure that an appropriate indication for ECT exists. A careful medical history and examination, focusing particularly on neurological, cardiovascular, and pulmonary systems, as well as upon effects of previous anesthesia inductions, are crucial to the establishment of the nature and severity of medical risk factors. To be sure that risk factors have been detected, their implications understood, and, where possible, mechanisms delineated for their correction or diminution, the patient should be evaluated prior to ECT by individuals privileged to administer ECT and ECT anesthesia.

Laboratory tests required as part of the pre-ECT workup vary considerably. In this regard, necessary procedures should be discriminated from those which are indicated only if positive findings on medical history, physical exam, or other laboratory tests suggest the need for further evaluation. A minimal screening battery of tests includes hematocrit and/or hemoglobin, serum electrolytes, and ECG. These procedures, along with the medical history and physical exam (including vital signs), will ensure that a basic evaluation of medical status has been carried out. Spine x-rays, now that risk of musculoskeletal injuries with ECT has been largely obviated by the use of muscular relaxation, are no longer considered necessary, unless pre-existing disease affecting the spinal columns is suspected or is known to be present. Likewise, EEG, brain computed tomography (CT), or magnetic resonance imaging (MRI) should only be considered if other data suggest that an abnormality may be present. The potential use of pre-ECT cognitive testing is discussed elsewhere (see Section 12.2).

The decision to administer ECT is based on the nature and severity of the patient's illness, treatment history, and a risk-benefit analysis of available psychiatric therapies, and requires agreement among attending physician, treating psychiatrist, and consentor. Medical consultation is sometimes used to obtain a better understanding of the patient's medical status, or when assistance in the management of medical conditions is desirable. To ask for "clearance" for ECT, however, makes the assumption that such consultants have the special experience or training required to assess both risks and benefits of ECT as compared to treatment alternatives—a requirement that is unlikely to be met. In some institutions, individuals in administrative positions make final decisions regarding the appropriateness of ECT. Such policies are inappropriate and compromise patient care.

10. Use of Psychotropic and Medical Agents During ECT Course

Medical agents. A review of all medications taken by the patient should be undertaken prior to initiation of the ECT course. Drugs prescribed for medical conditions are usually continued, although special attention is paid to anticonvulsants, lidocaine, and sedative/hypnotic agents, especially in the elderly. Since patients will receive various medications at the time of the ECT treatments themselves, drug-drug interactions should also be considered. Some antiarrhythmics, notably lidocaine and its recent analogs, raise seizure threshold (Hood and Mecca 1983), and substitutes should be considered. Theophylline increases the duration of seizures and heightens the likelihood of prolonged seizures (Peters et al. 1984; Devanand et al. 1988a). The increase in seizure duration by pretreatment with caffeine is the basis for its use in patients with very high seizure thresholds (see Section 11.8). Patients with glaucoma may continue their medications, unless they are receiving echothiopate or related agents with anticholinesterase properties, in which case they should be switched to alternative drugs. Some practitioners decrease dosage of anticonvulsant medications prior to ECT because of the known effects of such agents on seizure threshold, while others prefer to reduce dosage only if difficulty is experienced in producing adequate seizures.

An additional decision regarding concurrent use of medical pharmacologic agents with ECT is whether to administer the drugs before or after ECT on treatment days. In general, medications which exert a protective effect with respect to ECT-induced physiologic changes should be given prior to the treatment, usually, if in pill form, 1–2 hours earlier, with a sip of water. Examples include antiarrythmics (except lidocaine), antihypertensive, and antianginal agents, ventilatory stimulants (except theophylline), glaucoma medications (except anticholinesterases), and corticosteroids. In the latter case, even higher dosages may be indicated, due to the suppressive effects of long-term corticosteroid use. In diabetics, hypoglycemic medication, including insulin, is generally withheld until after the treatment, because of the patient's NPO status. With poorly controlled insulin dependent patients, the possibility of augmented blood glucose levels may necessitate increased insulin dosage during the ECT course (Finestone and Weiner 1984).

Psychotropic agents. For the most part, ECT is administered to patients who have not responded to prior trials of psychotropic medications. Except possibly for neuroleptic agents in the case of psychotic patients (see below), there is little justification at present for continuing these drugs during the ECT course, since evidence of synergistic action between ECT and most psychotropic agents has not been demonstrated (Seager and Bird 1962). Practitioners should be aware that abrupt discontinuation of many psychotropics, including antidepressant drugs as well as sedative/hypnotics, may produce withdrawal effects, and most such medications should be withdrawn on a stepwise basis.

There has been theoretical concern regarding the administration of anesthesia to patients receiving, or who have recently received, MAOI agents, although no evidence of untoward effects has been reported, despite extensive experience (Freese 1985; Remick et al. 1987; Wells and Bjorksten 1989). Lithium is usually discontinued prior to ECT because of potential toxicity. Patients receiving lithium during ECT appear to be at a higher risk for delirium, possibly as a result of greater brain levels of lithium produced by the increased permeability of the blood-brain barrier during ECT (Small et al. 1980; Strömgren et al. 1980; Standish-Barry et al. 1985; Rudorfer et al. 1987; el-Mallakh 1988; Ahmed and Stein 1987; Milstein and Small 1988). Benzodiazepines raise seizure threshold, reduce the duration of seizures, and may impair the efficacy of ECT (Strömgren et al. 1980; Standish-Barry et al. 1985; Pettinati et al. 1987; Nettlebladt 1988). Antipsychotic drugs may be continued during the course of ECT for psychotic or highly agitated patients, but are generally stopped after such symptoms remit. There are suggestive data that the combination of an antipsychotic drug with ECT may be more effective than ECT alone in psychotic patients (Smith et al. 1967; Friedel 1986; Gujavarty et al. 1987). The neuroleptic agent reserpine, now used primarily for its antihypertensive properties, has been associated with deaths when administered concurrently with ECT and should be avoided (Gaitz et al. 1956; Bross 1957).

11. Treatment Procedures

11.1. Preparation of the Patient

As described in Section 9, a pre-ECT psychiatric and medical evaluation should be completed prior to the first treatment. The treating psychiatrist should ensure that this evaluation is complete.

Prior to each treatment, nursing staff should ascertain compliance with pretreatment orders. Patients should have had nothing by mouth for at least six hours prior to the treatment, except for necessary medications with a small sip of water. Patients with cognitive impairment or psychosis may have difficulty in remembering restrictions on food and water intake and may require supervision. Nonetheless, when patients come to ECT they should be asked if they have taken anything by mouth over the past 6 hours. The nursing staff should ask patients to void and should check the head for pins and jewelry, and ensure that hair is clean and dry. The application of hair spray or hair creams is easily overlooked and can result in a shorting of the electrical current through the hair, resulting in singeing of the hair and failure to elicit a seizure. Eyeglasses, contact lenses, hearing aids, and dentures should be removed, unless there is a special indication (e.g., loose and isolated teeth may need protection). Vital signs should be recorded.

Prior to the treatment, the treating psychiatrist should check the treatment orders since the last ECT. Both the treating psychiatrist and anesthetist should be aware of any change in medications since the last treatment and any change in medical status. The patient's mouth should be checked for the presence of foreign bodies and loose or sharp teeth. When the patient is ready for ECT, intravenous access should be established. This usually involves maintaining an iv line with glucose or saline drip, although some practitioners prefer to inject medications directly into an indwelling catheter maintained with a heparin-lock. In either case, the iv line should be adequate to handle emergency needs, and care should be taken to ensure that all intravenously administered medications are followed by an infusion of vehicle. Intravenous access should be maintained at least until the patient is ready to leave the treatment area. Some practitioners prefer to leave the line in until the patient is ready to leave the recovery area, in case of delayed emergency. Particularly in patients in whom it is very difficult to establish iv access, some practitioners keep a heparin-lock in place between treatments. This procedure should be avoided, however, for patients at risk for pulling out the access either on purpose or inadvertently.

11.2. Airway Management

The anesthetist has responsibility for airway management throughout the ECT procedure. Prior to the first ECT of the day, the anesthetist should determine the adequate functioning of relevant equipment and the availability of supplies for resuscitation. The ability to ventilate the patient adequately should be determined prior to administration of the muscle relaxant. Patients with pulmonary disease or congestion may require particular attention. Unless there is a specific indication, use of intubation should be avoided.

Oxygenation (100% O_2, positive pressure, and a respiratory rate of 15–20 per minute) should be maintained from the onset of anesthesia until the resumption of adequate spontaneous respiration, except during application of the stimulus. Up to several minutes of preanesthetic oxygenation may be useful for patients with a history of myocardial ischemia. Oxygenation and ventilation prior to the application of the stimulus will help ensure that the elicited seizure is of adequate duration (Holmberg 1953; Chater and Simpson 1988; Räsänen et al. 1988). During the seizure, cerebral oxygen consumption increases on the order of 200% (Ingvar 1986). Maintaining oxygen delivery during the seizure will therefore aid in preventing hypoxia. Due to the effects of the muscle relaxant and the seizure, patients remain apneic during the immediate postictal state and require oxygenation until recovery of spontaneous respiration. Oximetry, to monitor adequacy of oxygenation, may be useful, particularly in patients in whom it is difficult to establish an adequate airway or who have pulmonary disease (see Section 11.7).

Prior to the application of the electrical stimulus, a flexible protective device ("bite-block") should be inserted in the mouth. The use of a Guedel-type plastic airway as a bite-block is not recommended because of increased risk of tooth fracture or jaw injury (Abrams 1988). The electrical stimulus results in direct stimulation of temporalis muscles and a clamping action of the jaw muscles which is not blocked by the muscle relaxant. To protect the teeth and other oral structures, the aim is to absorb the force of this clamping action by use of a flexible material that extends across the mouth, with maximal cushioning in the molar area. In uncommon instances of patients with only one or a few fragile teeth, use of a bite block may contribute to dental complications, and it may be preferable to leave dentures in place or to use gauze padding between the gums. During passage of the electrical stimulus, the patient's chin should be held up to keep the jaw tight against the bite-block so as to limit any potential trauma. The individual holding the patient's chin should not be in contact with an alternate ground path for the electrical stimulus, including the patient stretcher.

11.3. Medications Used with ECT

Anticholinergic agent. Immediately following the electrical stimulus there is frequently a short-lasting period of bradycardia which then converts to tachycardia with generalization of the seizure. Bradyrhythmia (e.g., atrial bradycardia) is also common during the postictal period. Premedication prior to anesthetic induction with a muscarinic anticholinergic reduces the risk of vagally mediated bradyrhythmias or asystole. There is limited evidence regarding the utility of such agents in moderating cardiovascular effects of ECT (Bouckoms et al. 1989; Miller et al. 1987; Rich et al. 1969; Wyant and MacDonald 1980) and not all practitioners routinely use such drugs. However, controlled studies largely excluded patients with pre-existing cardiac illness, limiting their relevance for patients believed to be at greatest risk for cardiovascular complications (Miller et al. 1987). Furthermore, if the electrical stimulus fails to elicit a seizure (subconvulsive), the bradycardia immediately following the stimulus is of graver concern, since the protection afforded by the ictal tachycardia (due to seizure-related catecholamine output) is absent, and there is a greater theoretical probability of asystole (Decina et al. 1984). Use of a muscarinic anticholinergic agent is specifically indicated for patients receiving sympathetic blocking agents or any other circumstance where it is medically important to prevent the occurrence of a vagal bradycardia.

Traditionally, such agents have been administered either intravenously 2–3 minutes prior to the anesthesia or, alternatively, intramuscularly or subcutaneously 30–60 minutes prior to anesthetic induction. The latter technique has the advantage of maximizing reduction of secretions, thereby potentially improving airway management. However, the intravenous route 2–3 minutes prior to the anesthesia is preferred by some practitioners, since it guarantees that the anticholinergic has been administered, obviates the need for an additional injection, and avoids increased dryness of the mouth at a time when the patient can not drink fluids. Perhaps most importantly, the action of the anticholinergic medication in increasing heart rate can be observed prior to the anesthetic induction, ensuring adequacy of anticholinergic dosage. Given individual differences in distribution and duration of action, intramuscular or subcutaneous administration 30–60 minutes prior to anesthesia may not offer protection in some cases.

The typical anticholinergic agents used are atropine 0.4–1.0 mg administered iv (or 0.3–0.6 mg administered im or sc) or glycopyrrolate 0.2–0.4 mg administered iv, im, or sc. Glycopyrrolate has the theoretical advantage of being less likely to cross the blood-brain barrier. However, controlled comparisons of glycopyrrolate and atropine in ECT have not revealed substantial differences in effects on cognition, cardiac function, or postictal reports of nausea (Greenan et al. 1985; Kellway et al. 1986; Swartz and Saheba 1989).

Anesthetic agent. ECT should only be performed using ultra-brief general anesthesia (Gaines and Rees 1986). The purpose of anesthesia is to have the patient unconscious during the seizure and the period of muscle relaxation. Therefore, the duration of unconsciousness should only last several minutes. Excessive anesthetic dosage may prolong unconsciousness and apnea, raise seizure threshold, shorten seizure duration, increase the risk of cardiovascular complications, and intensify amnesia. Consequently, the aim is to produce a "light-level" of anesthesia. However, if dosage is too light, loss of consciousness may be incomplete and autonomic arousal may occur.

Methohexital is presently the anesthetic agent preferred by most practitioners. Typical dose is 0.75–1.0 mg/kg given iv as a single bolus. Alternative agents are thiopental, etomidate, or ketamine. Thiopental may be associated with a higher incidence of postictal arrhythmias compared to methohexital (Pitts 1982). Ketamine may be associated with altered postictal states of consciousness, including hallucinations. Presently, propofol is not recommended as it may shorten seizure duration more than other agents. Regardless of the drug used, the adequacy of anesthetic dosage should be determined at each treatment so that dosage can be adjusted at subsequent treatments, as indicated.

Muscle relaxant. A skeletal muscle relaxant should be used to modify convulsive motor activity and to improve airway management. Before administration of the muscle relaxant, the anesthetist should ensure that a patent airway is present and that the patient will be unconscious prior to the onset of respiratory paralysis. The relaxant may be administered either immediately following the anesthetic agent or following initial signs of unconsciousness (the latter method is preferable at the first ECT because of uncertainty regarding adequacy of anesthetic dosage). Succinylcholine (0.5–1.0 mg/kg), by bolus or drip, is the preferred relaxant agent.

The purpose of the muscle relaxant is to produce sufficient modification of the convulsive movements to minimize the risk of musculoskeletal injury. Complete paralysis is neither necessary nor desirable. However, in some cases, such as patients with osteoporosis, a history of spinal injury, or with a pacemaker, complete relaxation may be indicated and dosage may be adjusted upward. Adequacy of muscle relaxation should be determined at each treatment session, with modification of dosages at successive sessions to achieve the desired effect. Atracurium and curare are alternative agents to succinylcholine.

Prior to application of the electrical stimulus, the adequacy of muscle relaxation is ascertained by determining the diminution or loss of knee, ankle, or withdrawal reflexes, loss of muscle tone, and/or by diminution or failure to respond to a nerve stimulator. A nerve stimulator is particularly useful for patients in whom extent of relaxation is uncertain and who are at heightened risk for musculoskeletal complications, and in whom non-depolarizing muscle relaxants such as curare or atracurium are used on an exclusive basis. With a depolarizing muscle relaxant such as succinylcholine, it is unlikely that maximal effect has taken place until after muscle fasciculations have disappeared.

Routine determination of pseudocholinesterase levels or of dibucaine number is not recommended. Such determinations should be reserved for patients with a personal or family history of prolonged apnea following exposure to muscle relaxants (Berry and Whittaker 1975; Viby-Mogensen and Hanel 1978). In the event of a positive test, or prolonged apnea at a previous treatment, very low doses of succinylcholine (e.g., 1–5 mg iv) or use of alternative agents, such as atracurium (e.g., 20–60 mg iv), should be considered. The anesthetist should be aware of the medical conditions and medications that may influence the action of muscle relaxant agents (Marco and Randels 1979).

After the first ECT, some patients report deep muscle pain. Particularly if the convulsive movements were well modified, this phenomenon may be due to intense fasciculations following succinylcholine administration. The intensity of succinylcholine-induced fasciculations may be diminished by administering curare (3–4.5 mg iv) or atracurium (3–4.5 mg iv) prior to the succinylcholine. If this is done, it may be necessary to increase the succinylcholine dose by 10%–25% to achieve the same degree of muscle relax-

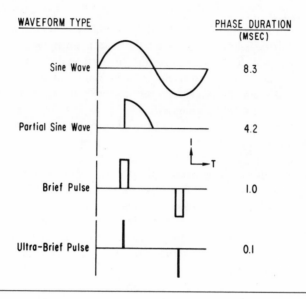

WAVEFORM TYPE

Sine Wave

Partial Sine Wave

Brief Pulse

Ultra-Brief Pulse

PHASE DURATION
(MSEC)

8.3

4.2

1.0

0.1

Figure 1. Examples of representative stimulus waveforms (repro-
duced with permission from Weiner 1982). A single cycle
of each waveform is shown, with current (I) on the
vertical axis, and time (T) on the horizontal.

ation as at the previous treatment, since succinylcholine and cura-
riform agents are competitive in their action.

11.4. ECT Devices

A variety of devices are available to administer ECT. For any
ECT device used, the nature and range of its stimulus parameters
and related features should conform to applicable national standards. A list of the devices presently marketed in the United States,
as well as a partial description of their features, is in Appendix D.
Reviews of device features are available (Nilsen et al. 1986; Stephens
et al. 1990). These devices generate either a unidirectional or
bidirectional pulse stimulus or a bidirectional sine wave stimulus.
Some ECT devices are capable of delivering more than one type of
waveform, as specified by the user. Figure 1 illustrates the waveforms
in present use, including some not presently available in the United
States. Waveforms differ in the intensity of stimulation needed to
produce seizures. Generally speaking, a more intense stimulus, in
units of charge (milliampere-seconds, mA-sec) or of energy (joules

or watt-sec), is necessary with a sine wave stimulus than with a brief pulse stimulus (Weiner 1980). This difference may be on the order of two- or three-fold. It is believed that the leading edge of each phase of the waveform is responsible for neuronal depolarization and seizure induction. Continuing to stimulate a neuron immediately after it has fired is inefficient, since there is a refractory period before it can again be depolarized.

As seen in Figure 1, the traditional sine wave stimulus is slow to reach maximum intensity and is long in phase duration. Therefore, at the beginning of each phase, stimulation is too low in intensity to produce effective depolarization. After peak intensity is reached with the sine wave, the long phase duration indicates that stimulation is likely administered during refractory periods. The brief pulse waveform reaches peak intensity virtually instantaneously (Figure 1). The duration of each pulse is short with virtual instantaneous return to baseline. Therefore, this configuration is more electrically efficient in eliciting seizures.

Comparative studies of sine wave and brief pulse waveforms have shown that cognitive side effects are more severe with sine wave stimulation (Weiner et al. 1986a). Likewise, there is evidence that disruption of the EEG is more profound with sine wave stimulation (Weiner et al. 1986b). These differences may be due to the greater electrical efficiency of brief pulse stimulation, or to other differences between the waveforms. In contrast, comparative studies have generally found that sine wave and brief pulse stimulation are equivalent in efficacy.

Two possible exceptions, however, should be noted. First, the use of ultra-brief pulses, i.e., pulses with durations less than 0.75–1.0 msec, may be associated with reduced efficacy (Cronholm and Ottosson 1963). Second, even with standard and longer duration pulses (1–2 msec), use of very low intensity stimulation, i.e., near the patient's seizure threshold, may reduce efficacy, particularly with a unilateral electrode placement (Sackeim et al. 1987b), or may require a longer course of treatments to achieve full response (Robin and de Tissera 1982).

ECT devices also differ in whether they operate on principles of constant current, constant voltage, or constant energy. With constant current devices, the peak current is either fixed or set by the user. The device adjusts the voltage administered during the stimulation to keep the current at the desired level. Voltage varies as a function of the impedance (or resistance) to the passage of the current. By Ohm's law (voltage = current × resistance), an increase in impedance requires an increase in voltage in order to keep the current constant.

Since the quality of contact at the interface between the electrodes and the skin is a major determinant of impedance, inadequate contact results in increased impedance. In such circumstances, constant current devices increase the output voltage so that the patient receives the predetermined stimulus current. Highly excessive output voltage may result in burns to the skin. For this reason, constant current devices should be equipped with voltage limiters, so that under abnormally high impedance conditions excessive voltage cannot be delivered. The user should be aware, however, that when the device limits the voltage due to too high impedance, current will not be maintained at the set level and the patient may fail to have a seizure or, if there is a seizure, the stimulus intensity may be close to threshold, with reduced therapeutic effects.

With constant voltage devices, the current varies inversely with impedance. By Ohm's law, an increase in impedance will result in a decrease in the intensity of the delivered current. It has been suggested that current intensity relative to the area of neural tissue through which it passes (current density) is the critical factor in both seizure induction and other neurobiological effects of the ECT stimulus (Sackeim et al. 1987c). Given this relationship, there is some concern about the rationale for the use of constant voltage principles in ECT devices. The user may not have access to information about the current intensity administered. In addition, with greatly increased impedance due to relatively poor contact or skin conditions, the resulting decrease in current intensity with constant voltage devices may be counterproductive in terms of ability to induce an adequate seizure.

Another approach to stimulus delivery is to keep the output energy constant. With such a device, the user selects the energy to be administered in units of joules (watt-sec). In order to keep the energy constant, the device will vary the duration of the stimulus. The theoretical justification for such a design is not self-evident. To deliver the user-determined energy, a shorter duration of stimulation will be administered in patients with high impedance than in patients with low impedance. Yet, as indicated earlier, it is unlikely that variation in impedance is relevant to therapeutic properties or adverse effects. Furthermore, doubt has been raised about the usefulness and validity of quantifying the ECT stimulus in units of energy (joules) as opposed to units of charge (mA-sec) (Sackeim et al. 1987c; Weiner et al. 1988).

Prior to the first use of an ECT device, the operator should establish familiarity with the principles that underlie operation of the apparatus. It is also important to ascertain and document that the stimulus output characteristics and all other controls, parameters, and features are functioning properly and are appropriately calibrated. Shipping and handling of the device can result in malfunction or miscalibration and users should not rely solely on the calibration performed by the manufacturer. The device manual provided by the manufacturer should outline the steps necessary to ensure adequate functioning, including the tolerance level for departure of parameters from exact values (e.g., ±10%).

As with other medical devices, a regular schedule of retesting or recalibration should be implemented, particularly in terms of electrical safety considerations. The intervals between retesting should minimally meet those stipulated in national standards, device manuals, and/or local facility requirements. The results of retesting should also be documented. Experience with ECT devices indicates that it is relatively rare to observe drift in stimulus output characteristics with standard use. However, if unusual conditions occur which may affect the integrity of the device (electrical malfunction, fire, spillage), immediate retesting should be carried out prior to subsequent clinical use.

There are several considerations regarding electrical safety in the administration of ECT. The ECT device should come equipped with a three-pronged, grounded electrical plug and must be connected to a three-pronged, grounded outlet approved for medical devices. Under no circumstances should the grounding be defeated, e.g., by plugging the device into a two-pronged outlet. Any electrical device in contact with the patient, unless battery operated, should be connected to the same electrical circuit as the ECT device. This may be accomplished by having all electrical equipment connected through the same power strip to an approved, grounded outlet.

Generally speaking, patient contact with other devices or other conducting media, such as metal bedrails, should be avoided, except when required for physiological monitoring. Contact of the patient with other devices or other conducting media increases the chances of alternative ground paths for the ECT stimulus. This is particularly likely if there is a ground fault in either device and both are not connected to the same power circuit. Under such conditions, a portion of the ECT stimulus current may pass through the heart, with potentially lethal effects. Likewise, for reasons of patient and staff protection, contact with the patient during the passage of the stimulus should be minimized. Under no circumstances should any individual other than the patient be in contact with the metal portion of the ECT electrodes during the passage of the stimulus.

The ECT device should be capable of use with either bilateral or unilateral electrode placement. This option will be ensured if stimulus cables, which connect to electrodes, are capable of independent movement. As described below, there is marked individual variability in the stimulus intensity that is needed to elicit adequate seizures (Sackeim et al. 1987c). Accordingly, the stimulus intensity controls on the device should allow the user sufficient flexibility to set stimulus intensity in relation to the needs of individual patients. Minimally, a device equipped with five incremental steps to regulate stimulus intensity may be acceptable, although more discrete control over stimulus intensity is advantageous. Given that some patients have a particularly high seizure threshold, it is recommended that brief pulse devices be capable of delivering at least 100 joules at a 220 ohm impedance. It may be that future devices should have higher intensity limits, dependent on the outcome of ongoing research.

For safety purposes, the device should indicate to the user that a stimulus is being delivered. Ordinarily this may be a tone and/or light that occurs only during the passage of current. The auditory mode is preferred by some practitioners as it does not require that the operator take his/her eyes off the patient during the initiation of stimulation. It is useful for devices to also be equipped with a distinct warning signal, to alert all members of the treatment team that a stimulus is about to be delivered. This feature helps to ensure that the stimulus is delivered only after preparation of the patient is complete and all staff involved in the procedure are ready. Likewise, for safety purposes, the ECT device should be equipped so that the user can abort the delivery of stimulus on an instantaneous basis if malfunction or other untoward events become apparent during the flow of the stimulus current.

11.5. Stimulus Electrode Placement

Electrode placement impacts on the extent and severity of cognitive side effects, with bilateral ECT associated with more short-term adverse effects than unilateral right (non-dominant) ECT (Sackeim et al. 1986a; Squire 1986). In some patients, electrode placement may also affect efficacy. In the treatment of major depressive disorders, most of the research literature finds that bilateral and unilateral right ECT are equivalent in short-term therapeutic effects (Fink 1979). However, when differences between the modalities have been observed, they have consistently favored bilateral ECT (Abrams 1986). When stimulus intensity is very low and just above seizure threshold the efficacy of unilateral right ECT is markedly reduced (Sackeim et al. 1987b). It has also been suggested that in manic patients bilateral electrode placement is particularly indi-

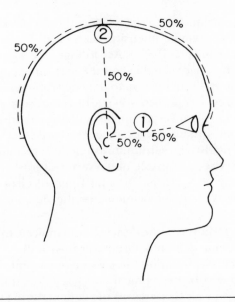

Figure 2. Location of stimulus electrodes with bilateral and right unilateral electrode placement. With bilateral ECT, stimulus electrodes are placed in position 1 on both sides of the head, with midpoints approximately one inch above the midpoint of a line between the tragus and the external canthus. With right unilateral ECT, one electrode is placed in position 1, while the other is located at position 2, at the intersection of the midpoints of lines going from left to right tragus and from inion to nasion.

cated (Small et al. 1986), although, this point is controversial (Mukherjee et al. 1988). In addition, there are reports of depressed patients who have shown poor response to unilateral right ECT subsequently responding to crossover treatment with bilateral ECT (Price and McAllister 1986), although there is also controversy in this regard (Strömgren 1984).

Given the intricacies involved in choice of bilateral versus unilateral ECT and their difference in side effect profiles, each facility should develop policies regarding use of unilateral and bilateral ECT. Of particular concern, the combination of bilateral electrode placement, high stimulus intensity, and sine wave stimulation is likely to maximize cognitive deficits without conferring additional therapeutic advantage. The determination of which electrode placement to use should, therefore, be made in concert with stimulus intensity considerations.

Some practitioners utilize unilateral or bilateral ECT exclusively. Others start depressed patients on unilateral ECT and switch to bilateral ECT if patients fail to respond or response is excessively slow (Abrams and Fink 1984). Another policy is to initiate bilateral ECT in patients for whom, on the basis of psychiatric or medical status, it is necessary to have greater guarantee of rapid clinical response. A further alternative strategy is to start all patients with bilateral ECT, switching to unilateral right ECT if cognitive side effects become severe, particularly in cases of sustained confusional state (organic brain syndrome).

Only one method of electrode positioning is in common use with bilateral ECT (bifrontotemporal position). The positioning involves estimating on each side of the head the midpoint of the line connecting the external canthus and the tragus. The midpoint of the stimulus electrode is then placed approximately one inch above this point (see Figure 2). A number of different placements have been used for unilateral ECT. A configuration that maximizes interelectrode distance may be optimal with regard to capacity to elicit seizures and efficacy (Pettinati et al. 1986). Among the unilateral placements, the d'Elia (1970) location is recommended. This placement involves determining the midpoint of an imaginary line connecting the two auditory tragi, running across the vertex of the scalp. The midpoint of the electrode is then placed approximately 1 inch lateral to this point (see Figure 2). A frontal unilateral placement should be avoided due to difficulties in seizure elicitation.

There is uncertainty about stimulus electrode placement in left handers. It has been estimated that approximately 70% of left handers are lateralized for language functions in a manner similar to that of right handers; 15% have bilateral representation of language and 15% have reversal of the typical pattern, with right hemisphere superiority for language functions (Bryden 1982). In right handers, unilateral right ECT produces less disruption of verbal functions than unilateral left ECT or bilateral ECT (Daniel and Crovitz 1983). The same should hold for the majority of left handers. One method that has been used to discern whether unilateral left or right ECT would be preferable, in order to avoid disruption to language functions, is to alternate the laterality of unilateral placement over the first few treatments to determine the placement associated with less severe acute confusion and verbal amnesia (Pratt et al. 1971) The possibility has also been raised that lateralization of function pertains to affective, as well as cognitive, realms (Sackeim et al. 1982). For instance, some data suggest that in most individuals the right hemisphere may play a greater role in the development and/or maintenance of depressed mood than the left. hemisphere. This hypothesis may account for some limited evidence that in treatment of depression unilateral right ECT is more efficacious than unilateral left ECT (Flor-Henry 1986), although these findings have recently been questioned; (Abrams 1989a; Abrams et al. 1989).

If handedness is taken into consideration in the determination of electrode placement, it is important to recognize that the hand used in writing and patient reports of handedness are fallible indicators. Many strongly left-handed individuals write with the right hand. Individuals who are basically right handed may report being ambidextrous or left handed (or vice versa) due to inconsistencies in hand usage for different activities. Inquiries should be made concerning a set of specific activities, such as throwing a ball, use of a knife and fork, use of scissors, etc. Standardized sets of items are readily available (e.g., Harris 1958). Predominant hand usage should determine assignment of handedness. Assessment of asymmetry in other domains (e.g., eyedness or footedness) is not germane.

Careful attention should be paid to preparation of the scalp at the sites of stimulus electrode placement and to the contact between electrodes and the scalp. Inadequate preparation and/or poor coupling results in increased impedance. With constant current devices, high impedance will result in the delivery of excess voltage or failure to maintain the current at the prescribed level. In the latter case, the patient may fail to have an adequate seizure (see Section 11.8) and the intensity of stimulation administered may be unknown. With constant voltage devices, this circumstance will produce a decrease in the intensity of current administered, also resulting in possible missed or abortive seizures.

A standard procedure should be developed at each facility regarding electrode site preparation. One method involves use of a solvent to cleanse the skin (ethyl acetate [nail polish remover] or acetone). After the site is dried, an abrasive conductant is rubbed into the scalp to lower site impedance. A conductant is then applied to the electrodes to ensure an adequate interface. If the electrode site is covered by a significant amount of hair, as is likely to be the case for the rostral (upper) electrode with unilateral placement, some practitioners have found it sufficient to simply part the hair prior to rigorous application of the solvent and conductant. Others find it advantageous to clip the hair at the site. If saline soaked pads are used as the conductant on electrodes, particular care must be taken that the saline is not dripped across the surface between electrodes. Indeed, smearing of any conducting medium between the electrodes will produce an alternate path for the stimulus current. This will result in the current passing across the scalp and not entering the brain, with consequent failure to elicit a seizure.

The electrodes should conform in size and composition to applicable national standards for ECT devices. Generally speaking, a larger electrode surface area will result in lower impedance to the passage of the current. The electrodes may be coupled to the scalp by use of a snugly fitting band or through the use of hand-held electrodes. Recently, adhesive pad electrodes have also been introduced. In general, firm pressure of the electrode against the scalp helps minimize impedance. Hand-held electrodes must be insulated so that the user is not in contact with the electrode or exposed wiring connecting the stimulus cable to the electrode. The use of tongs as electrode holders is discouraged. It is difficult to adjust tongs relative to asymmetries in skull anatomy, preventing proper electrode placement.

Some ECT devices are equipped to perform a "self-test" procedure prior to the administration of the stimulus. Use of such a procedure is strongly encouraged. During this procedure, an imperceptible current is passed, allowing determination of the integrity of the circuit. Specifically, the self-test procedure can be used to assess whether the impedance to the passage of this current is either too low or too high. The most common source of abnormally low impedance is smearing of a conductant medium between the electrodes. This may also result if the patient has administered a cream, gel, or spray to the hair, or has heavy perspiration. Too high impedance may be due to poor contact between an electrode and the scalp, incomplete or improper preparation of the electrode sites, poor contact between the electrodes and the stimulus cable, a break in the stimulus cable, or poor connection or disconnection of the stimulus cable from the device.

In the case of an abnormal self-test, the user should ascertain the cause of the low or high impedance problem and remedy it before proceeding with the treatment. Administration of another self-test procedure should determine whether the steps taken have been effective. In very rare circumstances, patients may have skin conditions that result in self-test abnormalities regardless of the integrity of the circuit. Some devices will explicitly alert the user to an abnormal self-test and will automatically disengage stimulus delivery. If it is believed that the self-test failure was due to intrinsic patient factors that can not be altered, these devices have override options so that stimulus delivery can be engaged despite the self-test failure. Other devices indicate to the user the impedance level determined from the self-test, without disengaging stimulus delivery. Devices that feature automatic disengagement of stimulus delivery therefore provide an extra margin of safety. In some cases where stimulation is given despite abnormally high impedance, the stimulus output may not match the parameters set by the user and the stimulus dose given to the patient will be unknown. It should be emphasized that with appropriate methods for electrode and scalp preparation and placement, administration of the stimulus despite an abnormal self-test should be an extremely rare event.

11.6. Stimulus Dosing

There is marked variability among psychiatric patients in the electrical threshold for eliciting an adequate seizure. This variability has been estimated to be as much as 40-fold (Sackeim et al. 1987c). If the same electrical intensity is used to elicit seizures in all patients, it must be extremely high to allow for patients with high thresholds. In patients with low thresholds, however, such a high intensity will be many times more than that needed to produce an adequate seizure, and may be associated with unnecessary cognitive side effects.

In considering dosage policy, two other factors need to be weighed. First, stimulus intensity may affect efficacy. Particularly with a unilateral non-dominant placement, stimuli barely above threshold may be therapeutically weak (Sackeim et al. 1987b). Regardless of electrode placement, speed of clinical response may be slower with barely suprathreshold stimuli than with moderately suprathreshold stimuli (Robin and de Tissera 1982). Second, the intensity of the ECT stimulus also affects short-term cognitive side effects. Higher intensity stimulation is associated with more severe deficits (Ottosson 1960).

Patients should receive stimulation that is moderately suprathreshold. Each facility should develop a policy on how this may be achieved. Until therapeutic windows are better defined, stimulus intensity 50%–200% above seizure threshold may be considered moderately suprathreshold. A dose 100% above threshold would require doubling (two times) the threshold dose, whereas 200% would involve tripling. It appears that efficacy with unilateral ECT may require a dosage that exceeds threshold to a greater extent than in bilateral ECT (Sackeim et al. 1987b).

In general, there are two approaches to determining stimulus intensity for individual patients. First, factors such as electrode placement, sex, age, anesthetic dosage, and concomitant medications impinge on seizure threshold. In relation to such factors, the practitioner may select a dosage for the first treatment that is empiricially suprathreshold for a sizable majority, e.g., 80% of patients. Second, some practitioners prefer to be cognizant of the degree to which stimulus dosage is suprathreshold. In this way they know with greater certainty whether they are delivering a moderately suprathreshold stimulus or one that is either minimally or excessively above threshold. To obtain such information, they may deliver an intensity at the first treatment that will elicit a seizure in only a minority of patients and then restimulate at successively higher intensities until a seizure is elicited (Sackeim et al. 1987c). In subsequent treatments, stimulus dosing may be adjusted to be moderately suprathreshold, based on the value established at the first treatment.

A policy concerning stimulus dosing should also consider that seizure threshold changes over the treatment course, with many patients manifesting large increases, e.g., 25%–200% (Sackeim et al. 1987d). Because of this phenomenon, dosage must generally be adjusted upwards to maintain a consistent suprathreshold level. In patients who show slow or inadequate clinical response and no more than mild cognitive side effects, an even further dosage increase may be considered. In patients for whom a level of stimulation has consistently produced adequate seizures and cognitive side effects are severe, a decrease of stimulus intensity may be considered and/or a switch to a unilateral nondominant placement or spacing of treatments over longer intervals.

Restimulation procedures following missed or abortive seizures are described in Section 11.8. The stimulus parameters administered and the number of stimulations should be documented at each treatment. There is no justification for continued use of glissando techniques, where the intensity of the stimulus is progressively increased during its delivery from a subconvulsive to convulsive level. Glissando was introduced prior to the use of general anesthesia in ECT as a means to produce unconsciousness (petit mal) and to prevent musculoskeletal injuries. With the introduction of general anesthesia, this technique is now only of historical interest.

11.7. Physiological Monitoring

Seizure duration. Each facility should develop a policy indicating criteria for the adequacy of seizure duration and how this will be determined (see Section 11.8). With few exceptions, seizures that are briefer than 20 seconds and seizures that do not bilaterally generalize (e.g., Jacksonian seizures) are believed to have reduced therapeutic properties. Yet, there are some patients who consistently fail to have seizures that exceed 20 seconds duration and, nevertheless, show clinical recovery with ECT. The duration of the seizure and the method of measurement should be documented at each treatment.

Perhaps the simplest and most reliable method of assessing seizure duration is by timing the duration of motor convulsive movements. However, these movements are much attenuated or absent with the use of muscle relaxants (succinylcholine). Therefore, it is recommended that distribution of such an agent to a distal portion of a limb (e.g., ankle or wrist) be blocked. Prior to administering the agent, a blood pressure cuff should be inflated to a pressure above the peak systolic pressure to be observed during the seizure (e.g., 250 mmHg). This procedure will allow for timing of unmodified convulsive movements without risk to the patient. It should be noted that even with such a procedure convulsive movements may be manifested for longer durations in other body regions, and the disappearance of all such movements should be taken as the endpoint.

If a unilateral electrode placement is used, the limb used should be on the same side as the electrode placement to ensure the ability to observe seizure generalization. Immediately following the seizure, the cuff should be deflated to prevent a prolonged ischemic period. Furthermore, particular care is necessary in use of this technique in patients at risk for musculoskeletal complications. For example, intense convulsive movements in the cuffed limb may cause fracture in patients with osteoporosis. Occasionally, patients may have adequate seizures that are not observed in terms of motor manifestations (Scott and Riddle 1989). This may be because the cuff is inflated too late, because the ictal pressure increase exceeds the restriction in circulation, or for other reasons. Also, patients rarely may have prolonged cerebral seizures or return of seizure activity (tardive seizures) that do not manifest in motor movements. For these reasons, it is strongly encouraged that in addition to observation of motor movements, seizures also be monitored with EEG.

At minimum, one channel of EEG activity should be monitored with either a paper record and/or auditory output. Prior to administration of anesthetic and muscle relaxing agents, the adequacy of the EEG record should be ascertained. The clinician should be familiar with the range of artifacts that may result in the EEG appearing to show seizure activity when none is present (anesthetic effects, movement, and ECG artifact, etc.) and the different manifestations of seizure termination. EEG monitoring should continue until the clinician is certain that seizure activity has terminated. This is most often indicated by a period of markedly attenuated activity following the high amplitude sharp and slow wave activity which occurs during the seizure.

If, for some reason, it cannot be determined whether or not a patient had a seizure, it may be useful to draw blood for prolactin determination during the period 10–30 minutes following stimulation. ECT-induced and spontaneous seizures produce a sharp rise in serum prolactin, e.g., 5- to 10-fold increase, over this time period (Abrams and Swartz 1985). Postictal peak values are generally in the 25–60 ng/ml range, whereas in patients not receiving neuroleptics, baseline values are typically below 10 ng/ml. If this procedure is done, it is important to obtain blood several hours after the treatment or the following day to make certain that the poststimulation value was markedly higher than the patient's baseline. If there is only a small difference between the two values, it is unlikely that the patient had a fully generalized seizure.

Cardiovascular monitoring. The morbidity and mortality associated with ECT are largely cardiovascular in origin. The period of greatest cardiovascular risk is between anesthetic induction and resumption of spontaneous respiration. Patients with history of cardiac illness are believed to present the greatest risk (Drop and Welch 1989; Prudic et al. 1987). Vital signs (blood pressure and pulse) and cardiac rhythms (ECG) should be monitored at frequent intervals from immediately prior to anesthesia administration until several minutes following seizure termination, or until there has been stabilization in these measures. Oscilloscopic or polygraphic monitoring of ECG is required, as transient postictal arrhythmias are often observed following the seizure, and occasionally may require intervention.

The capacity to provide a hard copy of the ECG should be readily available to document cardiac changes, to provide a more informed basis for consultation, and to assist in the management of complications at future treatments. Some ECT devices provide ECG hard copy output at non-standard chart speeds. If such output is entered in the patient's clinical records, the actual chart speed should be indicated or labelled timing marks provided. The anesthetist should be well aware of the variety of ECG changes observed during ECT, with an appreciation of those which usually do not require medical intervention (e.g., benign atrial arrythmia or PVCs), as opposed to those that typically require intervention (e.g., trigeminy, ventricular tachycardia).

Oximetry. Local standards of anesthetic practice may require routine use of pulse oximetry to assess adequacy of oxygenation. Regardless, oximetry may be valuable in patients with baseline ventilatory dysfunction, those in whom there is difficulty in maintaining an adequate airway, those who are at risk for prolonged apnea or seizures of long duration, or in patients with other conditions that raise the risk of hypoxia.

Safety considerations. For safety reasons described earlier, connection of an electrical monitoring device that is malfunctioning, particularly if there is a ground fault, can present a hazard to the patient. Further, the proper functioning of EEG, ECG, and oximetry devices is necessary to enhance the safety of the ECT procedure. Accordingly, prior to initial use, biomedical electronics personnel should be consulted to ensure the adequate functioning and safe use of physiological monitoring devices.

11.8. Management of Missed, Abortive, and Prolonged Seizures

Missed seizures. A "missed" seizure or subconvulsive stimulation occurs when, following electrical stimulation, there is no subsequent tonic or clonic seizure activity, although there may be a brief immediate contraction of some muscle groups in response to stimulation. The factors that lead to missed seizures include inadequate stimulus intensity, poor contact at the skin-electrode interface resulting in excessive dynamic impedance, hypercarboxia from inadequate ventilation, dehydration, and anticonvulsant action of medications (including benzodiazepines and barbiturate anesthetic agents).

Following a missed seizure, the practitioner should determine whether dynamic impedance was excessive, if such information is available. If the impedance value is excessive, the preparation of the electrode sites, adequacy of electrode position, and integrity of the electrical circuit should be examined and corrective measures taken. If excessive impedance was not at issue, the patient should be restimulated at higher stimulus dosage.

It is often preferable to wait 20–40 seconds between stimulations in the case of missed seizures. This is because some patients have delayed onset seizures. The delay may rarely be as long as 20 seconds or more. Secondly, the interval may also allow for dissipation of the effects of prior stimulation. An efficient treatment team will rarely need to administer additional anesthetic or muscle relaxing agents prior to restimulation, unless a large number of restimulations are required. It is common practice to restimulate at 25% to 100% above the original stimulus dosage.

In general patients should not leave the ECT suite failing to have had a seizure. There is some evidence that patients may experience prolonged confusional states following missed seizures. There may also be increased cardiovascular risk in administering a large number of subconvulsive stimulations over a short interval. Consequently, practitioners should carefully monitor cardiac status following missed seizures. Each facility should have a policy indicating the maximum number of subconvulsive administrations to be permitted prior to abandoning attempts to elicit a seizure at a treatment session, e.g., four or five.

Following the successful elicitation of a seizure, it is important to review the causes of the missed seizure, particularly when there is repeated difficulty in producing an ictal response. If possible, the patient's anticonvulsant medications should be reduced in dosage or discontinued. There is evidence that the dosage of barbiturate anesthetics is related to seizure threshold and duration, with larger doses increasing threshold and decreasing duration (Miller et al. 1985). The anesthetic dosage should be reviewed and possibly reduced. Vigorous hyperventilation should be attempted. Dehydrated patients should be examined for electrolyte imbalance with corrective measures taken. If the source of the problem is still not clear and increased stimulus intensity fails to elicit a seizure, then the practitioner may switch from a barbiturate anesthetic agent to ketamine (2 mg/kg iv) or use caffeine sodium benzoate as a pretreatment (500 mg to 2,000 mg iv, equivalent to 250–1,000 mg of pure caffeine) (Shapira et al. 1985, 1987; Coffey et al. 1987; Hinkle et al. 1987).

Abortive seizures. At times, seizures will be elicited that are abortive, that is, too short in duration, typically less than 20–30 seconds by EEG criteria. If, for instance, a policy is adopted that adequate seizures must be 20 seconds in duration, a 12-second seizure would be considered inadequate. In such circumstances, procedures similar to those following a missed seizure should be implemented. The same factors that are responsible for missed seizures can produce abortive seizures. Abortive seizures, however, may be due to either insufficient stimulus intensity or excessive stimulus intensity. There is evidence that when stimulus dosage is barely above seizure threshold some patients may have weak, abortive seizures. Increasing intensity will increase seizure duration. However, other data suggest that markedly suprathreshold stimulation may decrease seizure duration (Robin et al. 1985). Therefore, too low or too high stimulus parameters may produce abortive seizures and the practitioner may need to estimate where on the intensity versus seizure duration curve they are likely to be.

Following an abortive seizure, there is likely to be a sharp transient increase in seizure threshold. Restimulation immediately after an abortive seizure will often produce a missed seizure or another abortive seizure, due to this threshold increase. To partially overcome this "refractory period," it is advisable to use a longer time interval prior to restimulation than in the case of a missed seizure. Some practitioners have found an interval of 60–90 seconds sufficient. In addition, some practitioners believe that the increase in stimulus intensity may need to be higher for restimulation following an abortive seizure, relative to a missed seizure. Prior to restimulation, the patient should be examined to determine whether or not there is a need to administer additional anesthetic and muscle relaxant agents., e.g., return of spontaneous respiration or of consciousness. As in the case of missed seizures, the possible causes of abortive seizures should be reviewed prior to the next treatment session, with particular attention to factors that may increase seizure threshold. A common cause of both missed and abortive seizures is excessive dose of the anesthetic agent.

In determining whether patients have had an adequate treatment, some practitioners calculate total seizure time from multiple stimulations. There is no empirical justification for this practice. A patient who has had two abortive seizures in a session, each of 11 seconds, should not be considered to have had an adequate treatment because the total seizure time exceeded a 20-second criterion. However, it should be emphasized again that regardless of the adequacy of technique, some patients consistently display short seizures (e.g., 18 seconds in motor manifestations). This is particularly likely to occur later in the ECT course, since seizure duration declines and seizure threshold rises with progressive treatment (Sackeim et al. 1986b). There is no evidence that such patients do not benefit from these treatments. In contrast, the concern about abortive seizures centers on the patient who is capable of manifesting a fully adequate seizure, but has one of short duration due to factors such as concomitant medication, inadequate ventilation, inadequate or excessive stimulus intensity, or poor electrical contact.

Prolonged seizures. Rarely, some patients experience prolonged seizures following ECT or may have a return of seizure activity after the initial seizure terminates (tardive seizures). A prolonged seizure is defined here as one greater than 3 minutes in duration. Each facility should develop a set of procedures describing the steps to be taken in response to such events.

EEG monitoring can be invaluable in such cases, as prolonged or tardive seizure activity may not be expressed in motor movements. Maintenance of an adequate level of oxygenation may require intubation if the seizure is grossly prolonged or if there is evidence of hypoxia. Usually after 3 minutes of seizure activity, the seizure should be aborted pharmacologically. Administration of the same barbiturate anesthetic agent (e.g., methohexital) at the same dosage used for ECT anesthesia usually terminates the seizure. Intravenous administration of single, and if neccesary, repeated doses of a benzodiazepine, e.g., diazepam (5–10 mg) or midazolam (1–2 mg) is also likely to be successful.

Patients should be monitored closely during this period, particularly for cardiovascular crisis, with monitoring continuing until return of consciousness and stable vital signs. After stabilization of the acute situation, further evaluation may be advisable to determine the cause of the prolonged seizure, the steps that may be useful to prevent recurrence, and the presence of any sequelae. A decrease in stimulus intensity at subsequent treatments should be considered following a prolonged seizure, unless such a dosage previously resulted in a missed or abortive seizure. The practitioner should be familiar with the circumstances that are likely to give rise to prolonged or tardive seizures, as described in Section 4.

11.9. Postictal Recovery Period

Physiological monitoring should continue until patients are ready to be transferred from the treatment area to the recovery room. Patients should not be released from the treatment area until spontaneous respiration has resumed with adequate tidal volumes and return of pharyngeal reflexes, vital signs and ECG are stable so that patient can return to a lower level of observation, and there are no adverse effects requiring immediate medical evaluation or intervention. Patients should be brought by stretcher or bed to the recovery area.

Management of patients in the recovery area should be supervised by the anesthetist, who should be readily available in case of emergency. The recovery nurse should provide continuous observation and supportive care. Patients should be gently reoriented. Vital signs should be assessed at least at 15-minute intervals starting with arrival in the recovery area. Patients are ready to leave the recovery area when awake with stable vital signs and otherwise

102 The Practice of Electroconvulsive Therapy

prepared to return to ward care or to the care of responsible significant others (if outpatients). Prior to departing from the recovery area, the recovery nurse should inquire about nausea, headache, or other adverse states. The ward staff or significant others should be informed of special conditions or the need for additional monitoring or supervision. For inpatients, the patient should be fed after leaving the recovery area.

Postictal delirium. Some patients develop a postictal delirium or excitement, characterized by motor agitation, disorientation, and poor response to commands. Recovery may take from 5 to 45 minutes, usually with amnesia for the episode. Postictal delirium may result in physical injury due to the patient thrashing against hard objects. In addition, patients may dislodge the intravenous line, complicating management. Depending upon severity, postictal delirium may be managed supportively or pharmacologically. If supportive intervention is used, the patient should be gently re-strained to protect against physical injury and intravenous line loss and should be continuously reassured. Too firm restraint may aggravate the condition. Pharmacological management typically involves iv administration of the agent used to produce anesthesia or a benzodiazepine sedative/hypnotic agent (e.g., diazepam or midazolam). Such agents should be administered after return of spontaneous respiration, and, if possible, prior to the patient leaving the treatment area. Suggested starting doses are 20 mg of methohexital, 2.5–5 mg of diazepam, or 0.5–1 mg midazolam, with readministration as needed.

Postictal delirium may be observed at one or more ECT treatments in approximately 10% of patients (Devanand et al. 1989). It may occur at a single treatment, never to recur, or it may occur at each treatment in the course. Prophylaxis is recommended when it is believed that the postictal delirium is recurrent, by observation at more than two consecutive treatments. Prophylaxis involves administering the anesthetic agent or benzodiazepine prior to the emergence of the syndrome, but after the return of spontaneous respiration.

11.10. Frequency and Number of Treatments

In the United States, ECT is most commonly performed at a schedule of three times per week regardless of electrode placement. Some practitioners have suggested administration of unilateral ECT at a schedule of 5 treatments per week in the belief that more frequent treatment may speed recovery. Some practitioners also believe that daily use of ECT, regardless of electrode placement, may be useful early in the treatment course when a particularly rapid response is necessary, as in cases of severe mania, catatonia, high suicidal risk, or severe inanition. Prolonged use of daily treatments or use of more intense regimens (e.g., regressive ECT) should be avoided due to heightened risk of cognitive dysfunction. A reduction in the frequency of treatment should be one of the methods considered if severe cognitive dysfunction or delirium develops.

Psychiatric patients vary widely in the number of treatments necessary to achieve a full clinical response. The total number administered should be a function of both the patient's degree and rate of clinical improvement and the severity of cognitive adverse effects. For those patients who achieve clinical remission, the treatment course should terminate as soon as it is evident that maximal improvement has been reached. There is no evidence that additional treatment of the acute phase beyond that necessary to achieve remission impacts on rate of relapse (Snaith 1981). Termination of ECT should also be considered in patients who have shown substantial but not full clinical improvement, but who remain unchanged after two more treatment sessions.

Evaluation of response should focus on changes in target symptoms, with assessment made between each ECT treatment. While the typical ECT course in mood disorder patients is between 6 and 12 treatments, some patients manifest complete remission after only a few treatments. Other patients may not begin to show substantial clinical change until they have received 10 or more treatments (Sackeim et al., 1990). Larger numbers of treatments may be needed when a change in ECT technique has taken place due to lack of response, and also in some cases of schizophrenia. In patients with slow or minimal clinical improvement, the indication for continued ECT should be reassessed after 6–10 treatments. At such time, consideration may be given to modification of ECT technique. The changes to consider include switching from unilateral to bilateral ECT, increasing stimulus intensity levels, and using medications to potentiate the ictal response or otherwise augment efficacy (e.g., addition of a neuroleptic with psychotic patients).

Each facility should have a policy regarding the number of treatments that may be given before a formal assessment of the need to continue ECT is documented. The recommendation to administer additional ECT should be discussed with the consentor (Section 5.3), as well as other changes in treatment that may substantially impact on risk/benefit considerations.

Repeated courses of ECT are sometimes necessary due to relapse or recurrence of the psychiatric condition. The decision to readminister a course of ECT within a six-month period should take into account the quality of the previous response to the treatment, including occurrence of adverse effects. In particular, the presence and severity of persistent cognitive deficits should be considered, especially if bilateral electrode placement had been previously used or will be used in the upcoming course (Weiner et al. 1986a).

There is no evidence that repeated courses of ECT lead to permanent structural damage (Weiner 1984), or that a maximum limit on lifetime number of treatments with ECT is needed. However, frequent relapses should suggest that present attempts at continuation or maintenance therapy are ineffective (Sackeim et al., in press). In patients who require repeated treatment of acute episodes with ECT, attention should be given to the adequacy of post-ECT pharmacotherapy in terms of the type, dosage, and duration of medication. If standard pharmacotherapy trials are ineffective in preventing relapse, or if adequate pharmacotherapy cannot be tolerated by the patient due to side effects, consideration should be given to use of ECT as a continuation or maintenance treatment (see Section 13).

Some practitioners have advocated calculating cumulative seizure time across treatment sessions, with the suggestion that a time duration window should be used in determining whether or not the patient has received a sufficient number of treatments (Maletzky 1968). More recent studies suggest that this practice is not valid (Weiner et al. 1986b; Sackeim et al. 1987b).

11.11. Multiple Monitored ECT

Multiple monitored ECT (MMECT) is a form of treatment in which more than one adequate seizure is produced under continuous anesthesia in the same treatment session. Proponents of this technique suggest that a smaller number of treatment sessions, and therefore a shorter time interval, is required to produce the same quality of remission as with conventional ECT (Maletzky 1981). Critics of the method contend that MMECT is associated with a higher risk of neurological morbidity and adverse cognitive effects (Abrams 1988). Although a substantial minority of practitioners in the United States currently use MMECT on at least an occasional basis, controlled comparisons of MMECT and conventional ECT have yet to be reported. Some practitioners reserve use of MMECT to patients who have a high anesthetic risk or an urgent need for rapid onset of therapeutic response. Others limit the number of seizures in a treatment session to two.

Facilities that provide MMECT should specify the procedures that must be followed in its use. This includes requiring both EEG and ECG monitoring, stipulating the recommended intervals between seizures within a treatment session and between treatment sessions, limiting the maximum number of adequate seizures to be elicited per treatment session, and limiting the maximum number of electrical stimulations to be applied. Since seizure duration increases with repeated induction during the same treatment session (Maletzky 1981), it is particularly important that the policy and procedures for managing prolonged and tardive seizures be defined. The requirement with MMECT of a continuous period of anesthesia also indicates that procedures for how this is to be accomplished should be specified. This includes the type, method of administration, and dose ranges of anesthetic agents and muscle relaxants. Information describing the known or likely differences in the benefits and risks of MMECT, compared to conventional ECT, should be provided to the consentor when use of this technique is considered.

11.12. Outpatient ECT

ECT may be performed on an outpatient basis provided that there has been careful selection of suitable patients and the facility is properly equipped and staffed to do so. Facilities that provide outpatient ECT should monitor adherence to the special policies that pertain to use of this treatment on an outpatient basis.

In selecting patients for outpatient ECT, the same indications, contraindications, consent requirements, and pre-ECT evaluations as described above apply. In addition, the patient's psychiatric condition should not present a contraindication to management on an outpatient basis. For example, patients with suicidal intent should not be treated as outpatients. Psychotic patients raise doubt as to capacity to follow instructions regarding behavioral limitations and should not be treated as outpatients. Likewise, patients who present with anticipated risks that are not likely detectable or manageable during the ECT session or on an outpatient basis should be excluded. Examples include patients at increased risk to develop a post-ECT delirium (e.g., pre-existing neurological impairment, history of ECT-induced organic brain syndrome) or patients with medical complications that increase the risks of ECT (e.g., unstable aneurysm).

Patients selected for outpatient ECT should be willing and able to comply with the required behavioral limitations over the time period of the treatment course and immediately thereafter. It is strongly encouraged that patients have available a significant other who will assist in ensuring compliance with these behavioral limitations. An attending physician should be designated to maintain overall responsibility for patient management during and immediately following the outpatient ECT course. This individual should be available for consultation with the patient, pertinent significant others, and the ECT treatment team. The treating psychiatrist may be so designated. Since the patient's condition may change with time, his/her suitability in meeting these criteria should be reevaluated on an ongoing basis.

Patients and significant others should be informed that the patient must follow a set of behavioral limitations. The use of a written instruction sheet is encouraged, but does not take the place of formal discussion with a member of the ECT treatment team. These instructions should be conveyed prior to the start of outpatient ECT, with reinstruction and reminders on a regular basis. Compliance with behavioral limitations should be assessed prior to each treatment.

Patients should avoid activities that are likely to be impaired by the adverse cognitive effects of ECT. Since there are marked individual differences in the severity and longevity of cognitive side effects, and since these adverse effects also vary with treatment parameters, limitations on activities should be tailored to individual patients and adjusted as indicated. With long intervals between treatments, as is typical with continuation or maintenance ECT, adverse cognitive side effects usually do not persist beyond the day of the treatment. At minimum, patients receiving outpatient ECT as a treatment for an acute psychiatric condition should be specifically instructed to refrain from making major life decisions until completion of the ECT course and clearing of residual cognitive side effects. This includes matters pertaining to business, personal finances, and interpersonal relations. Patients should also be instructed to refrain from driving during the acute course. Patients and significant others should be instructed to inform the attending physician and/or the ECT treatment team of any changes in medical condition or of adverse effects of ECT. This information should be conveyed as soon as possible, and certainly before the next treatment. Explicit instructions should be given regarding dietary regimens to be followed prior to each treatment, as well as bowel, bladder, and grooming behavior. At each treatment, it is important to check prior to induction of anesthesia that dietary instructions have been followed. In addition, patients and pertinent significant others should be instructed about the importance of abiding by medication regimens, including any adjustments to be made on the day of each treatment.

Prior to each outpatient ECT, it is particularly important for the treatment team to check compliance with instructions regarding oral intake, voiding, cleanliness and dryness of hair, and removal of dentures and other foreign bodies from the mouth. The treating psychiatrist should ascertain whether any unexpected or severe adverse effects took place following the previous treatment, whether any change in medical conditions or alteration in medication regimen or compliance has occurred over the interval between treatments, and whether any further evaluation or alteration in treatment technique is indicated.

It is suggested that facilities providing outpatient ECT have a space near the recovery or treatment areas in which outpatients and family members can wait prior to release from the facility. Outpatients should be released from the recovery area to this waiting area. Observation in the waiting area may be provided either by the facility's nursing staff or by the patient's significant other. Standards for release of outpatients from the facility should be stricter than the criteria for release of inpatients from the recovery area to the ward. Outpatients will usually have to return to home and they should be capable of independent locomotion and of negotiating traffic. It is preferable that outpatients be accompanied by family or friends when released from the facility, and facilities should consider making this a requirement. If this procedure is not followed, a member of the treatment team or designee should evaluate psychomotor and cognitive status prior to release from the facility. Functioning should be compatible with a safe journey home without assistance.

12. Evaluation of Outcome

12.1. Therapeutic Response

Prior to the start of ECT, each patient should have a documented treatment plan, indicating specific criteria for remission. Prominent symptomatology should be described in terms of type and severity. It is helpful for therapeutic goals to take into account which aspects of symptomatology are expected to improve. For example, some mood disorder patients present with chronic dysthymia prior to emergence of a full blown episode of major depression. In the context of ECT, there is no empirical evidence as to whether remission of a major depressive episode is associated with return to the chronic dysthymia or whether dysthymic symptomatology also improves. However, some practitioners believe that dysthymic symptoms do improve and that focusing treatment termination on resolution of the major depressive episode alone may result in incomplete treatment, with possible heightened risk of relapse. In contrast, some patients with schizoaffective disorder present with relatively chronic forms of thought disorder (e.g., delusions), upon which is superimposed prominent episodic affective symptomatology. In a number of these patients, ECT may ameliorate the affective component without influencing the chronic thought disorder. Prolonging the ECT course to attempt such resolution may result in unnecessary treatment.

After the start of ECT, clinical assessments should be performed by the attending physician or designee after every one or two treatments. These assessments should preferably be conducted on the day following a treatment to allow for clearing of acute cognitive effects and should be documented. The assessments should include attention to changes in the episode of mental disorder for which ECT has been referred, both in terms of improvement in signs and symptoms present initially and the manifestation of new ones. During the course of ECT, switches from depression to mania may occur on an uncommon basis. In this context, it is important to distinguish between an organic euphoric state and mania (Devanand et al. 1988b) (see also Section 11.9). Formal assessment of changes in cognitive functioning may help in making this differential diagnosis.

In patients treated for prominent catatonic symptomatology, the nature of other symptoms may have been difficult to discern at pretreatment due to mutism or negativism. With introduction of ECT and the clearing of catatonia, other aspects of psychopathology may become evident and should be assessed and documented. Some patients may have experienced delusions or hallucinations prior to or during the ECT course, but, due to patient guardedness or other factors, these symptoms may have been difficult to verify. With clinical improvement, the clinician may ascertain their presence, a determination which may impinge on discharge planning and future treatment.

12.2. Adverse Effects

Cognitive changes. The impact of ECT on mental status, particularly regarding orientation and memory functioning, should be assessed both in terms of objective findings and patient report during the ECT course (see Section 4). This assessment should be conducted prior to the start of ECT in order to establish a baseline level of functioning and repeated at least weekly throughout the ECT course. It is suggested that cognitive assessment, like assessment of therapeutic change, be conducted at least 24 hours following an ECT treatment to avoid contamination by acute postictal effects.

The evaluation may include either bedside assessment of orientation and memory and/or more formal test measures. It should include determination of orientation in the three spheres (person, place, and time), as well as immediate memory for newly learned material (e.g., reporting back a list of three to six words) and retention over a brief interval (e.g., reporting back the list 5–10 minutes later). Remote recall might likewise be assessed by determining memory for events in the recent and distant past (e.g., events associated with the hospitalization, memory for personal details— address, phone number, etc.).

Formal testing instruments provide quantitative measures for tracking change. To assess global cognitive functioning, an instrument such as the Mini-Mental State exam (Folstein et al. 1975) may be used. To track orientation and immediate and delayed memory, subtests of the Russell revision of the Weschler Memory Scale could be used (Russell 1988). To formally assess remote memory, tests of recall or recognition of famous people or events can be used (Butters and Albert 1982; Squire 1986). When cognitive status is assessed, the patient's perception of cognitive changes should also be ascertained. This may be done by informally inquiring whether the patient has noticed any changes in his/her abilities to concentrate (e.g., to follow a television program or a magazine article) or to remember visitors, events of the day, or recall of more remote events. Patient perception of memory functioning may also be examined using a quantitative instrument (Squire et al. 1979).

In the event that there has been a substantial deterioration in orientation or memory functioning during the ECT course that has not resolved by discharge from the hospital, a plan should be made for post-ECT follow-up of cognitive status. Most commonly there is marked recovery in cognitive functioning within days of the end of the ECT course (Steif et al. 1986) and patients should be reassured that this will likely be the case. The plan should include a description of when follow-up assessment would be desirable, as well as the specific domains of cognitive function to be assessed. It may be prudent in such cases to conduct additional evaluations, e.g., neurological and electroencephalographic examinations, and if abnormal to repeat until there is resolution.

It should be kept in mind that the cognitive evaluation procedures suggested here provide only gross measures of cognitive
status. Furthermore, interpretation of changes in cognitive status
may be subject to a number of difficulties. Psychiatric patients
frequently have cognitive impairments prior to receiving ECT and
a therapeutic response may therefore be associated with improvement in some cognitive domains (Sackeim and Steif 1988). However, while some patients show improved scores relative to their
pre-ECT baseline, they still may not have fully returned to their
baseline level of cognitive functioning (Steif et al. 1986). This
discrepancy may be a basis for complaints about lingering cognitive
deficits. In addition, the procedures suggested here only sample
limited aspects of cognitive functioning, for example, deliberate
learning and retention of information. Patients may also have
deficits in incidental learning. Likewise, the suggested procedures
concentrate on verbal memory, although both right unilateral and
bilateral ECT produce deficits in memory for nonverbal material
(Squire 1986).

Other adverse effects.   During the ECT course, any onset of new
risk factors, or significant worsening of those present at pre-ECT,
should be evaluated prior to the next treatment. When such devel-
opments alter the risks of administering ECT, the consentor should
be informed and the results of this discussion documented. Patient
complaints about ECT should be considered adverse effects. The
attending physician and/or a member of the ECT treatment team
should discuss these complaints with the patient, attempt to determine their source, and ascertain whether corrective measures are
indicated.

13. Management of Patient's Post-ECT Course

Continuation therapy, which is defined as the extension of somatic
therapy over the 6-month period following induction of a remission
in the index episode of mental illness, has become the rule in
contemporary psychiatric practice. Exceptions may include patients
who are intolerant to such treatment and possibly those with either
an absence of prior episodes or a history of extremely long periods
of remission (although compelling evidence for the latter is lacking). Unless residual adverse effects necessitate a delay, continuation therapy should be instituted as soon as possible after remission
induction, since the risk of relapse is especially high during the first
month. Some practitioners believe that the onset of symptoms of

impending relapse in patients who are ECT responders may represent an indication for institution of a short series of ECT treatments for a combination of therapeutic and prophylactic purposes, although controlled studies are not yet available to substantiate this practice.

Continuation pharmacotherapy. A course of ECT is usually completed over a 2- to 4-week period. Standard practice, based in part on earlier studies (Seager and Bird 1962; Imlah et al. 1965; Kay et al. 1970), and in part on the parallel between ECT and psychotropic drug therapies, suggests continuation of unipolar depressed patients with antidepressant agents (with the possible addition of an antipsychotic drug in cases of psychotic depression), bipolar depressives with antidepressant and/or antimanic medications; and manics with antimanic and possibly antipsychotic agents. For the most part, dosages are maintained at 50%–100% of the clinically effective dose range for acute treatment, with adjustment up or down depending upon response. Still, the role of continuation therapy with psychotropic drugs after a course of ECT is undergoing assessment, and our recommendations should be considered provisional. Disappointment with high relapse rates, especially in patients with psychotic depression and in those who are medication resistant during the index episode (Sackeim et al., 1990), compels reconsideration of present practice, including a renewed interest in continuation ECT (Fink 1987b).

Continuation ECT. While psychotropic continuation therapy is the prevailing practice, few studies document the efficacy of such use after a course of ECT, and some recent studies report high relapse rates even in patients complying with such regimens (Spiker et al. 1985; Aronson et al. 1987, 1988a, 1988b; Sackeim et al., in press). These high relapse rates have led some practitioners to recommend continuation ECT for selected cases. Recent retrospective reviews of this experience find surprisingly low relapse rates among patients so treated, although controlled studies are not yet available (Kramer 1987; Decina et al. 1987; Clarke et al. 1989; Löo et al. 1988; Matzen et al. 1988; Thornton et al. 1988).

Because continuation ECT appears to represent a viable form of continuation management of patients following completion of a successful course of ECT, facilities are encouraged to offer this modality as a treatment option. Patients referred for continuation ECT should meet all of the following criteria: 1) history of recurrent illness that is acutely responsive to ECT; 2) either refractoriness or intolerance to pharmacotherapy alone or a patient preference for

ECT; and 3) the ability and willingness of the patient to receive continuation ECT, provide informed consent, and comply with the overall treatment plan, including any behavioral restrictions that are necessary.

Because continuation ECT is administered to patients who are in clinical remission, and because long inter-treatment intervals are used, many facilities offer it on an outpatient basis (see Section 11.12), if this is logistically feasible (see Section 8). The specific timing of treatments with continuation ECT has been the subject of considerable discussion, but evidence supporting any set regimen is lacking at present. In many cases, treatments are started on a weekly basis, with the interval between treatments gradually extended to a month, depending upon the patient's response. Such a plan is designed to take into account the high likelihood of early relapse noted earlier. In general, the greater the likelihood of early relapse, the more intensive the regimen should be. For the most part, psychotropic agents are not used during a series of continuation ECT. Still, because of the refractory nature of many such cases, some practitioners supplement continuation ECT with such medication in selected cases, particularly in those who are not well controlled on continuation ECT alone.

Before each continuation treatment, the attending physician should make a full assessment of clinical status, inter-treatment experience and symptoms, and should make a determination that the treatment is indicated. Documentation of the further need for continuation treatment should be made periodically, no longer than every 3 months. Informed consent should be renewed no less frequently than every 6 months (see Section 5). In order to provide an ongoing assessment of risk factors, an interval medical history and physical exam, focussing on specific systems at risk with ECT, should be done prior to each treatment. In many settings this brief evaluation is accomplished by the treating psychiatrist and anesthetist on the day of the treatment. Full physical exams and laboratory tests (see Section 9) should be repeated at least every 3 months, and the ECG no less frequently than annually. Since cognitive effects with continuation ECT appear to be less severe than with the more frequent treatments occurring during an ECT course, assessment of cognitive function (see Section 12) may be done as infrequently as every 3 treatments.

Continuation psychotherapy. For some patients, individual and/or group therapy may be useful in dealing with underlying psychodynamic issues (particularly in cases of secondary depression), in facilitating better ways to cope with stressors that might otherwise precipitate a clinical relapse, in assisting the patient to re-organize his/her social and vocational activities, and in encouraging a fuller return to normal life.

Maintenance therapy. Maintenance therapy, empirically defined as the prophylactic use of psychotropics and/or ECT longer than 6 months past induction of a remission in the index episode, is indicated when attempts to stop continuation therapy have been associated with symptom recurrence, when continuation therapy has been only partially successful, or when a particularly strong history of recurrent illness is present. The specific criteria for maintenance ECT, as opposed to maintenance psychotropic therapy, are the same as those described above for continuation ECT. The frequency of maintenance ECT treatments should be kept to the minimum compatible with sustained remission (usually one treatment every 1–3 months), with re-evaluation of the need for extension in the treatment series and repeated application of informed consent procedures performed at the intervals listed above for continuation ECT.

14. Documentation

A patient's medical record is a legal document. It provides evidence for what did or what did not take place in his or her contact with the health care facility. Information contained in the medical record also helps members of the clinical management team to provide safe, effective, and efficient care. In addition, such information facilitates later evaluation and treatment. Finally, documentation assists with quality assurance and utilization review activities. Still, it must be understood that, while adequate documentation is essential to modern medical practice, time spent writing in the medical record is no substitute for time spent in direct patient care activities. For this reason, documentation should be kept at a level which facilitates quality of care rather than hampers it. In this regard, except for complex situations, notes in the clinical record should be concise and to the point, with detail limited to essential material.

Because the medical record represents the primary source of all clinically related information, the facility's medical director should maintain overall responsibility for assuring that adequate documentation is achieved.

A course of ECT is not begun until a proper pre-ECT evaluation has taken place, relevant risks and benefits assessed, informed consent completed, and a treatment plan adopted. Documentation of this process helps to ensure that it has been completed in an appropriate fashion and that potential problems have been considered. While much of such documentation is usually provided by the attending physician, it is the responsibility of the treating psychiatrist, who is in charge of the administration of the ECT treatments, to ensure that necessary documentation is in order prior to the first treatment and each successive treatment.

In terms of specific areas for documentation, it is important to address why a referral for ECT has been made and to delineate relevant risk/benefit considerations. Since the determination of treatment endpoint is based upon an appreciation of baseline symptomatology, major target symptoms and their severity should be noted prior to treatment onset. Similarly, the ongoing assessment of adverse effects requires a baseline determination of orientation and memory function (see Section 12.2).

The signing of a formal consent document prior to ECT is required in virtually all jurisdictions within the United States. In addition, a summary of major consent-related discussions should also be included in the medical record (see Section 5). Such a summary should include, but not be necessarily limited to, a description of and justification for ECT in situations associated with substantial alterations in indications, risks, and/or treatment technique, and a description of procedures undertaken in cases of limited or absent capacity to consent.

The clinical record should demonstrate that the clinical management team is aware on an ongoing basis of the presence or absence of both therapeutic change and adverse effects over the ECT course. At a minimum, weekly notes containing such information will suffice, although more frequent entries are optimal. Adverse effects occurring during the time the patient is in the treatment and recovery areas should also be documented. When an ECT treatment course is unusually prolonged (see Section 11.10), or a series of continuation/maintenance treatments is extended for an additional 3-month period (see Section 13.3), reasons for these actions should be briefly described in the clinical record.

It is good clinical practice and, for that matter, good common sense, to document the essential parameters of the treatment procedure at the time of each ECT treatment. The availability of such information helps the treatment team to administer successive treatments in a safe and effective fashion, assists future caregivers in the determination of proper treatment parameters, and is useful for ongoing quality assurance purposes. In many facilities, members of the ECT treatment team rotate on a weekly or even daily basis, rendering such data particularly important.

Specific treatment information to be documented include: electrical stimulus parameters, stimulus electrode placement type, seizure duration, all medications given in the treatment and recovery room (including dosage), and vital signs (e.g., blood pressure and pulse). As with any procedure requiring general anesthesia, the anesthetist should provide a brief note covering the patient's condition while in the treatment area. Similarly, the recovery area staff should document vital signs and orientation while the patient is under their care. Any substantial adverse effects occurring in the treatment or recovery areas should likewise be summarized in the clinical record, including actions taken and recommendations made regarding future management.

In addition to information entered into the clinical record, it is also useful to keep a separate record within the treatment area itself of treatment parameters and medications given. Such material is helpful, not only in case the data contained in the clinical record is lost, but also because it provides a means to easily reconstruct how the ECT was administered even months or years later, e.g., when the patient returns with a recurrence of illness. Again, documented material of this type also facilitates quality assurance and utilization review activities.

Just as it is important to document the rationale for beginning an ECT course or series, it is also helpful to provide a basis for the decision to end the course or series of treatments. Typical reasons for stopping ECT include achievement of maximal clinical benefit, failure to respond therapeutically after an adequate trial, adverse effects (type and severity should be noted), and patient refusal. Since the risk of relapse following a course of ECT or, for that matter, following completion of an acute phase of treatment with psychopharmacologic agents, is high (see Section 13), a plan for continuation management should be documented. When indicated, follow-up plans for assessment and/or treatment of adverse effects present at time of discharge should also be briefly noted, including a short description of these effects, as well as how and by whom they will be monitored.

15. Education and Training in ECT

Contrary to what some may believe, ECT has evolved into a highly technical and complex treatment (Fink 1986). Major technical advances, directed towards maximizing efficacy and minimizing risks, have occurred in instrumentation for stimulus delivery, stimulus electrode placement, pharmacologic modification of induced seizures, and physiological monitoring. While such advances have gone a long way towards optimizing risk-benefit considerations, they have come at the cost of substantially greater training needs. The traditional training venue of observation followed by trial (and error) is most certainly inappropriate in the present setting. Unfortunately, requirements for more intense training in ECT come at a time when utilization of this treatment has diminished and training demands for other treatments has increased.

In this regard, present training in ECT in many residency programs ranges from marginal to totally absent—a situation which must be corrected to ensure that future generations of practitioners are able to deliver ECT in a safe and effective fashion (Fink 1986). Recent surveys of ECT practice done outside of the United States point out only too clearly the dangers associated with inadequate training (Pippard and Ellam 1981; Anonymous 1981). Department chairmen, residency training directors, and departmental faculty as a whole should recognize that certain minimal training requirements (see below) should be considered a prerequisite for the establishment of clinical competency. Likewise, those responsible for providing privileging in ECT (see Section 16) should take care to set a high priority upon the training background of those seeking such privileges.

The practice of ECT is multidisciplinary, and involves professionals trained in psychiatry, anesthesiology, and nursing. In addition, other medical specialists are frequently called upon to provide consultative services to patients being evaluated for ECT, or find themselves caring for patients who either are receiving or recently have had exposure to this treatment modality. Because the treating psychiatrist is the leader of the ECT treatment team and therefore requires comprehensive knowledge of ECT-related topics, the training curriculum in ECT within psychiatric residency programs requires a substantial time commitment. While coverage of anesthetic considerations for ECT are considerably more narrow in their focus and therefore less time consuming, anesthesiology and nurse anesthetist training programs should not ignore this material entirely. Finally, in addition to medical school, residency, and nursing school training, there is a need for ongoing Continuing Medical Education (CME) opportunities in ECT, to help ensure a continued level of competence by practitioners and to provide a means by which those whose training is otherwise deficient can attain the level of educational experience required for clinical privileging in ECT.

Medical school. Brief, but comprehensive, didactic coverage of ECT should be included as part of the psychiatric training experience in medical school. It is suggested that at least one hour be spent on such topics. Given the rather substantial degree of misinformation about ECT to which medical students may have already been exposed, adequate time for student discussion should be provided. Medical students should be encouraged to observe ECT practice either directly or via videotape. Efforts should be made to monitor the quality of medical school education in ECT. On a national level, the National Board of Medical Examiners should incorporate a reasonable coverage of ECT-related topics in Part II of their examination.

Psychiatry residency.   In order to accomplish training goals for psychiatry residency programs, it is important that department chairmen and residency training directors set a priority on the development of adequate curricula (including making sure that qualified faculty are chosen to be involved in the program). These individuals should also monitor the program's adequacy on an ongoing basis and take measures to ensure that deficiencies are corrected. It is understood that not all departments have faculty who are sufficiently well qualified in ECT to be responsible for teaching such courses. In such cases, arrangements should be made to bring in outside practitioners for this purpose.

In terms of the didactic portion of the ECT curriculum in residency training programs, it is important that there be an opportunity for interchange between faculty and trainees, so that questions can be answered and views clarified. Accordingly, although video tape material is often a useful supplement to didactic instruction (see Appendix C), there should not be an exclusive reliance on such aids.

There has been considerable variability in the type and amount of didactic instruction on ECT provided in psychiatry residency training programs. Although some programs provide formal lecture or seminar presentations, others incorporate ECT-related material into curricula for other aspects of psychiatry, e.g., psychopharmacology or affective disorders. Still other programs appear to make the assumption that practical experience in ECT will somehow provide any information that might otherwise be covered in a didactic format. This practice is ill founded. The didactic curriculum should cover all major aspects of the ECT procedure, including mechanisms of action, selection of patients, risks and adverse effects, pre-ECT evaluation, informed consent, methods of administration, evaluation of therapeutic outcome, management of patients following completion of an ECT course (including the potential role of continuation/maintenance ECT), and malpractice considerations. Alternative viewpoints should be reflected in areas that are marked by present controversy.

The amount of time necessary to cover the above material will vary, but a minimum of four hours is required to give a good overview, while allowing a sufficient opportunity for discussion. Programs that are unable to provide at least this much time for ECT should take explicit steps to make sure that remaining topics are covered within the context of practical experience in ECT (see below), rather than simply assuming that this process will take care of itself.

Although important, didactic teaching is clearly insufficient to provide all training necessary to administer ECT. As noted earlier, the practice of ECT is a highly technical and sophisticated medical procedure. Accordingly, didactic instruction must be supplemented by an intensive, well-supervised practical training experience. Unfortunately, it has been traditional in some psychiatric training settings for residents, usually in the first and second years of their program, to be responsible for providing delivery of ECT with little or no supervision. It is also not rare for supervision, when present, to be provided by members of the faculty who themselves may be poorly trained and lacking in demonstrable skills. This situation is deplored and should not be tolerated by residency programs. Efforts should be made to ensure the presence of direct supervision by the most highly qualified individuals available, even if such personnel must be secured from outside the department. To further the teaching impact of practical training in ECT, the use of teaching materials such as assigned readings, videotapes, etc., should be encouraged.

The amount of practical experience in ECT necessary to allow development of adequate skills will vary from resident to resident, as well as from program to program. At a minimum, a resident should participate in the administration of at least 10 ECT treatments, each directly supervised by a psychiatrist privileged in ECT. To provide exposure to differing case material, at least three separate cases should be included in the series. These minimal requirements represent a trade-off between what is optimally desirable and what is feasible in many training programs.

A 1976 survey involving the American Association of Directors of Psychiatric Residency Program undertaken by a previous APA Task Force recommended approximately twice this number of treatments (American Psychiatric Association 1978). Similarly higher requirements were reported recently in Denmark (Bolwig 1987). However, a recent survey of the directors of 23 psychiatry residency training programs in the United States revealed that most respondents believe that a minimum of two to five patients should be administered ECT by residents during their training (Yager et al. 1988). To an extent, these latter views may well be based upon an appreciation of the variable amount of ECT case material that is presently available in teaching institutions. For that matter, in a recent survey of medical schools, approximately 20% of respondents indicated that ECT was not used at all in the primary teaching hospitals (Raskin 1986).

In addition to the actual administration of ECT, residents should gain experience in the clinical management of patients undergoing an ECT course, including the pre-ECT evaluation, informed consent, and choices of type, number, and frequency of ECT treatments, as well as post-ECT management. As a minimum, each resident should actively participate in the care of at least two such patients. Practical experience in the evaluation and case management of ECT patients is particularly important, given the fact that a much larger number of psychiatrists are presently involved in providing such care than are involved with the direct administration of ECT. A recent large survey of psychiatric practitioners, department chairmen, and training directors reflects the view that knowledge about case management of patients receiving ECT is considered a more important component of the general psychiatric training experience than are skills gained in the actual administration of this treatment modality (Langsley and Yager 1988).

These recommendations for didactic and practical training in ECT are viewed as constituting minimal requirements, and residency programs should be encouraged to exceed these levels. The use of clinical case conferences, ECT rounds, and elective opportunities for advanced training in ECT represent particularly useful ways to increase the quality of the overall learning experience. Still, it is understood that some residency training programs, particularly those in settings where the practice of ECT is minimal or even absent, may simply not have sufficient resources available to meet these requirements. In such cases, attempts should be made to cover as much of the above curriculum as possible, making use of assigned readings, videotaped material, and outside speakers. Residents in such programs should be explicitly told that supplementation of their training experience will be required before they should consider themselves competent to administer ECT on an unsupervised basis.

To ensure that ECT training in psychiatry residency programs is adequate, the specific educational and training experiences offered by the program should be documented. In addition, programs should evaluate residents' performance in the ECT-related components of the curriculum. Records of such evaluations should be kept for purposes of ongoing program evaluation and for use as credentials in the ECT privileging process (see Section 16). In line with policies already implemented for some medical and surgical procedures, psychiatry residents should be encouraged to keep records of both ECT treatments administered by them, as well as of patients under their care who have received ECT (taking appropriate measures to ensure confidentiality). Such information is also useful in helping to satisfy ECT privileging requirements.

Anesthesiology residency. Anesthesiology residency programs should incorporate specific training in ECT into their curricula. It should not be assumed that general education and training in anesthesia will suffice. It is particularly important that areas where ECT anesthesia differs from standard anesthetic practice be covered in depth. The physiological changes accompanying the electrically induced seizure, for example, represent a normal part of the ECT procedure and not a cause for alarm and institution of emergency corrective action. In addition, doses of anesthetic agents used for procedures other than ECT may be so high as to make it difficult to produce adequate seizures with ECT or may complicate postictal recovery.

Training in ECT for anesthesiology residents should be provided by qualified individuals, including faculty involved in the ECT training of psychiatric residents. As with psychiatry residents, training in ECT for anesthesiology residents should include both didactic and practical training components. In terms of the didactic exposure, a concise, though comprehensive, perspective should be provided, including a discussion of ECT's role in contemporary psychiatric practice. There should be an in-depth coverage of areas of specific anesthetic interest. Such topics include the pre-ECT evaluation, use of medications during the ECT procedure, pertinent drug interactions, provision of oxygenation (including the effects of hyperventilation upon the ictal response), use of physiological monitoring, physiological and behavioral effects of the post-ictal state, and electrical safety considerations. Again, sensitivity to areas where ECT anesthesia differs from standard practice should be given particular attention. Major adverse effects that may occur in treatment and recovery areas should also be enumerated and their management discussed. Just as it is important that psychiatric residents receive adequate supervision in ECT, anesthesiology residents should likewise be supervised by qualified individuals while taking part in their own practical training experience.

Nursing. As nursing personnel are important members of the ECT treatment team, education in ECT should be provided as part of the nursing school experience. In terms of didactic instruction, a general overview of ECT should be provided, supplemented by an in-depth focus upon areas where nursing personnel are likely to play a major role (see Section 7). As with all aspects of ECT training, instruction should be provided by qualified individuals, making use wherever possible of those involved in actual clinical administration of ECT. Opportunity for observation of ECT administration is useful, either directly or through use of videotaped material. Post-graduate training for psychiatric nursing administrators should include additional instruction and training in ECT. The curricula for nurse anesthesia programs should incorporate the material described above for anesthesiology residents.

Specialty boards. Regardless of professional discipline, one means of helping to ensure that adequate training has been provided is for specialty boards to require exposure to education and/or training in ECT for board eligibility. Precedents for such a requirement for other procedures have already been considered by boards in medical and surgical specialties. At the least, specialty boards in psychiatry, anesthesiology, and nursing should incorporate a representative number of questions on ECT into their examinations.

Continuing medical education. As noted earlier, continuing medical education (CME) opportunities allow practitioners to keep their knowledge and skills up to date as well as providing a means to help those who are deficient in their educational and training backgrounds to gain credentials for clinical ECT privileging (Fink 1986). Participation in such programs is particularly important for psychiatrists, but is also useful for anesthesiologists and nurses. Attendance at CME programs can and should be an important factor in the maintenance of ECT privileges (see Section 16).

Although a number of excellent CME programs have been offered, there is clearly room for many more, particularly with respect to practical education and training. Professional organizations should take the initiative in encouraging the development and implementation of such programs at annual meetings and elsewhere. Symposia, courses, seminars, and fellowship opportunities in ECT at the local, regional, and national levels should be publicized widely. A particular need exists at present for opportunities offering hands-on training in ECT, as very few ongoing formal programs exist at the time of the writing of this document (see Appendix C). For this reason, many clinicians presently rely upon informal arrangements, which are often less satisfactory from an educational perspective.

16. Privileging in ECT

Throughout these guidelines, it has been made clear that provision of safe and effective ECT requires the involvement of competent staff (see especially Section 7). How best to ensure the clinical competency of staff involved in the administration of ECT has been the subject of considerable discussion. The determination of clinical competency of practitioners is usually handled by certification and/or privileging. No national board provides certification specifically for ECT. Accordingly, assurance of clinical competency of practitioners is presently provided in the form of local privileging. In practice, clinical privileges for a given specialty, subspecialty, or procedure are granted by a facility's medical director to applicants who meet specific educational, training, experience, and skill criteria set by the facility's organized medical staff. The materials provided by the applicant in this process constitute his or her credentials. Staff members must also reapply to maintain privileges, usually at regular intervals. In this way, each facility, through a peer review process, ensures that its clinical services are provided in as safe and effective a fashion as possible. Often, privileging covers practice of an entire discipline, e.g., psychiatry, anesthesia, etc. In recent years, however, because of the growing level of technical sophistication involved in clinical practice as well as a heightened sensitivity to quality of care considerations, there has been a trend toward greater specificity in privileging practices. Given the extent of knowledge and skill required to administer ECT, it is quite clear that general privileging in psychiatry will not suffice and that specific clinical privileges to administer ECT should be required.

Privileges to administer ECT should be granted only to psychiatrists who meet formal, documented criteria set by the organized medical staff. The facility's medical director should establish that these criteria are met prior to an applicant's administration of ECT on an unsupervised basis. The medical director should use qualified personnel to assist with this determination, including outside consultants as appropriate. The candidate's education, training, experience (including history of past ECT privileging), and demonstrated skill should be the specific determinants in the granting of ECT privileges. Medical licensure, satisfactory completion of residency training, and board certification or eligibility, should be considered in addition to ECT-related material such as evidence of satisfactory completion of relevant residency and CME training experiences, and letters of recommendation. The extent of training and experience required should at least be sufficient to satisfy the educational and training recommendations described in Section 15.

To help establish the presence of adequate skills in the administration of ECT, the applicant should be observed in the delivery of ECT, and should demonstrate sufficient skill to satisfy the privileging authority. The individual evaluating the applicant's clinical skills should be a psychiatrist who is already privileged in ECT. Should no such person be available in the facility, provisions should be made for the use of an outside consultant. In cases where an applicant's education, training, and/or skills in ECT are deficient, further training should be required. This training experience should consist of didactic instruction and/or individualized reading, as well as a formal or informal clinical practicum, if indicated. Decisions as to the scope and depth of the training program should be guided by the type and degree of deficiencies present. Should skills in administering ECT be assessed as inadequate, the recommended training should include provision by the applicant of at least 10 ECT treatments under supervision, in order to ensure that at least the minimum practical training requirements of Section 15 have been met. Following satisfactory completion of the training program, the applicant should still be required to demonstrate proficient administration of ECT in the facility granting privileging.

Each facility granting privileges for ECT should also devise policies and procedures to maintain such privileges. This practice is required to ensure that a sustained level of clinical competence can be achieved. The plan for maintenance of privileging should make use of ongoing quality assurance programs, as well as the monitoring of individual practice patterns, especially the number of treatments administered yearly. Any evidence of deficiencies in practice should be corrected immediately. The plan should also include a requirement for CME in ECT-related areas. Reapplication for clinical privileges should be made at least every two years, or as otherwise specified by regulation or by general local policies covering clinical privileging. The plan should include a provision for reassessment of clinical skills for individuals whose practice of ECT has been inactive for a considerable time, e.g., one year.

Problems occur when a facility is so small that it does not have an organized medical staff, or when the facility does not have sufficient expertise to adequately evaluate applications for ECT privileging. In such situations, the existence of concurrent clinical privileges obtained from a separate facility may be an acceptable substitute, although an attempt should be made to institute procedures for formal in-house privileging as soon as possible, involving the use of outside consultants as deemed necessary.

Bibliography

Abrams R: Is unilateral electroconvulsive therapy really the treatment of choice in endogenous depression? Ann NY Acad Sci 462:50–55, 1986

Abrams R: Electroconvulsive Therapy. New York, Oxford University Press, 1988

Abrams R: Lateralized hemispheric mechanisms and the antidepressant effects of right and left unilateral ECT. Convulsive Therapy 5:244–249, 1989a

Abrams R (ed): ECT in the high risk patient. Convulsive Therapy 5:1–122, 1989b

Abrams R, Fink M: The present status of unilateral ECT: some recommendations. J Affective Disord 7:245–247, 1984

Abrams R, Swartz CM: ECT and prolactin release: effects of stimulus parameters. Convulsive Therapy 1:38–42, 1985

Abrams R, Taylor MA: Unipolar and bipolar depressive illness: phenomenology and response to electroconvulsive therapy. Arch Gen Psychiatry 30:320–321, 1974

Abrams R, Taylor MA: Catatonia: a prospective clinical study. Arch Gen Psychiatry 33:579–581, 1976

Abrams R, Swartz CM, Vedak C: Antidepressant effects of right versus left unilateral ECT and the lateralization theory of ECT action. Am J Psychiatry 146:1190–1192, 1989

Addonizio G, Susman VL: ECT as a treatment alternative for patients with symptoms of neuroleptic malignant syndrome. J Clin Psychiatry 48:102–105, 1987

Ahmed SK, Stein GS: Negative interaction between lithium and ECT. Br J Psychiatry 151:419–420, 1987

Alexander RC, Salomon M, Ionescu-Pioggia M, Cole JO: Convulsive therapy in the treatment of mania. Convulsive Therapy 4:115–125, 1988

Allen RE, Pitts FN Jr: ECT for depressed patients with lupus erythematosus. Am J Psychiatry 135:367–368, 1978

Allen RM: Pseudodementia and ECT. Biol Psychiatry 17:1435–1443, 1982

Allman P, Hawton K: ECT for post-stroke depression: beta blockade to modify rise in blood pressure. Convulsive Therapy 3:218–221, 1987

American Psychiatric Association Task Force on ECT: Electroconvulsive Therapy. Task Force Report No. 14. Washington, DC, American Psychiatric Association, 1978

American Psychiatric Association: Diagnostic and Statistical Manual of Mental Disorders, Third Edition. Washington, DC, American Psychiatric Association, 1980

American Psychiatric Association: Diagnostic and Statistical Manual of Mental Disorders, Third Edition, Revised. Washington, DC, American Psychiatric Association, 1987

Ananth J, Samra D, Kolivakis T: Amelioration of drug-induced Parkinsonism by ECT. Am J Psychiatry 136:1094, 1979

Andersen K, Balldin J, Gottfries CG, Granérus AK, Modigh K, Svennerholm L, Wallin A: A double-blind evaluation of electroconvulsive therapy in Parkinson's disease with "on-off" phenomena. Acta Neurol Scand 76:191–199, 1987

Anonymous: ECT in Britain: a shameful state of affairs [editorial]. Lancet 2:1207–1208, 1981

Applebaum PS, Lidz CW, Meisel A: Informed Consent: Legal Theory and Clinical Practice. New York, Oxford University Press, 1987

Aronson TA, Shukla S, Hoff A: Continuation therapy after ECT for delusional depression: a naturalistic study of prophylactic treatments and relapse. Convulsive Therapy 3:251–259, 1987

Aronson TA, Shukla S, Hoff A, Cook B: Proposed delusional depression subtypes: preliminary evidence from a retrospective study of phenomenology and treatment course. J Affective Disord 14:69–74, 1988

Assael MI, Halperin B, Alpern S: Centrencephalic epilepsy induced by electrical convulsive treatment (abstract). Electroencephalogr Clin Neurophysiol 23:195, 1967

Atre-Vaidya N, Jampala VC: Electroconvulsive therapy in parkinsonism with affective disorder. Br J Psychiatry 152:55–58, 1988

Avery D, Lubrano A: Depression treated with imipramine and ECT: the DeCarolis study reconsidered. Am J Psychiatry 136:559–562, 1979

Avery D, Winokur G: Mortality in depressed patients treated with electroconvulsive therapy and antidepressants. Arch Gen Psychiatry 33:1029–1037, 1976

Avery D, Winokur G: The efficacy of electroconvulsive therapy and antidepressants in depression. Biol Psychiatry 12:507–523, 1977

Avery D, Winokur G: Suicide, attempted suicide, and relapse rates in depression. Arch Gen Psychiatry 35:749–753, 1978

Bagadia VN, Abhyankar RR, Doshi J, Pradhan PV, Shah LP: A double blind controlled study of ECT vs chlorpromazine in schizophrenia. J Assoc Physicians India 31:637–640, 1983

Balldin J, Edén S, Granërus AK, Modigh K, Svanborg A, Walinder J, Wallin L: Electroconvulsive therapy in Parkinson's syndrome with "on-off" phenomenon. J Neural Transm 47:11–21, 1980

Balldin J, Granërus AK, Lindstedt G, Modigh K, Walinder J: Predictors for improvement after electroconvulsive therapy in parkinsonian patients with on-off symptoms. J Neural Transm 52:199–211, 1981

Baxter LRJ, Roy-Byrne P, Liston EH, Fairbanks L: Informing patients about electroconvulsive therapy: effects of a videotape presentation. Convulsive Therapy 2:25–29, 1986

Berman E, Wolpert EA: Intractable manic-depressive psychosis with rapid cycling in an 18-year-old woman successfully treated with electroconvulsive therapy. J Nerv Ment Dis 175:236–239, 1987

Berry M, Whittaker M: Incidence of suxamethonium apnoea in patients undergoing E.C.T. Br J Anaesth 47:1195–1197, 1975

Bibb RC, Guze SB: Hysteria (Briquet's syndrome) in a psychiatric hospital: the significance of secondary depression. Am J Psychiatry 129:224–228, 1972

Black DW, Wilcox JA, Stewart M: The use of ECT in children: case report. J Clin Psychiatry 46:98–99, 1985

Black DW, Winokur G, Nasrallah A: The treatment of depression: electroconvulsive therapy v antidepressants: a naturalistic evaluation of 1,495 patients. Compr Psychiatry 28:169–182, 1987a

Black DW, Winokur G, Nasrallah A: Treatment and outcome in secondary depression: a naturalistic study of 1,087 patients. J Clin Psychiatry 48:438–441, 1987b

Black DW, Winokur G, Nasrallah A: Treatment of mania: a naturalistic study of electroconvulsive therapy versus lithium in 438 patients. J Clin Psychiatry 48:132–139, 1987c

Blackwood DH, Cull RE, Freeman CP, Evans JI, Mawdsley C: A study of the incidence of epilepsy following ECT. J Neurol Neurosurg Psychiatry 43:1098–1102, 1980

Bolwig TJ: Training in convulsive therapy in Denmark (letter). Convulsive Therapy 3:156–157, 1987

Bouckoms A, Welch C, Drop L, Dao T, Kolton K: Atropine in electroconvulsive therapy. Convulsive Therapy 5:48–55, 1989

Brandon S, Cowley P, McDonald C, Neville P, Palmer R, Wellstood-Eason S: Electroconvulsive therapy: results in depressive illness from the Leicestershire trial. Br Med J 228:22–25, 1984

Brandon S, Cowley P, McDonald C, Neville P, Palmer R, Wellstood-Eason S: Leicester ECT trial: results in schizophrenia. Br J Psychiatry 146:177–183, 1985

Breakey WR, Kala AK: Typhoid catatonia responsive to ECT. Br Med J 2:357–359, 1977

Bross R: Near fatality with combined ECT and reserpine. Am J Psychiatry 113:933, 1957

Bruce EM, Crone N, Fitzpatrick G, Frewin SJ, Gillis A, Lascelles CF, Levene LJ, Mersky HA: A comparative trial of ECT and Tofranil. Am J Psychiatry 117:76, 1960

Bryden M: Laterality: Functional Asymmetry in the Intact Brain. New York, Academic Press, 1982

Bulbena A, Berrios GE: Pseudodementia: facts and figures. Br J Psychiatry 148:87–94, 1986

Burke WJ, Rutherford JL, Zorumski CF, Reich T: Electroconvulsive therapy and the elderly. Compr Psychiatry 26:480–486, 1985

Butters N, Albert M: Processes underlying failures to recall remote events, in Human Memory and Amnesia. Edited by Cermak L. Hillsdale, NJ, Erlbaum, 1982, pp 257–274

Carr ME Jr, Woods JW: Electroconvulsive therapy in a patient with unsuspected pheochromocytoma. South Med J 78:613–615, 1985

Carr V, Dorrington C, Schrader G, Wale J: The use of ECT for mania in childhood bipolar disorder. Br J Psychiatry 143:411–415, 1983

Casey DA: Electroconvulsive therapy in the neuroleptic malignant syndrome. Convulsive Therapy 3:278–283, 1987

Chang SS, Renshaw DC: Psychosis and pregnancy. Compr Ther 12:36–41, 1986

Chater SN, Simpson KH: Effect of passive hyperventilation on seizure duration in patients undergoing electroconvulsive therapy. Br J Anaesth 60:70–73, 1988

Clarke TB, Coffey CE, Hoffman GW, Weiner RD: Continuation therapy for depression using outpatient electroconvulsive therapy. Convulsive Therapy 5:330–337, 1989

Clinical Research Centre, Division of Psychiatry: The Northwick Park ECT trial: predictors of response to real and simulated ECT. Br J Psychiatry 144:227–237, 1984

Coffey CE, Weiner RD, Hinkle PE, Cress M, Daughtry G, Wilson WH: Augmentation of ECT seizures with caffeine. Biol Psychiatry 22:637–649, 1987

Consensus Conference: Electroconvulsive therapy. JAMA 254:2103–2108, 1985

Constant J: Treatment of delirious episodes. Rev Prat 22:4465–4473, 1972

Corsellis JAN, Meyer A: Histological changes in the brain after uncomplicated electroconvulsive treatment. Journal of Mental Science 100:375–383, 1954

Cronholm B, Ottosson J: Ultrabrief stimulus technique in electroconvulsive therapy, II: comparative studies of therapeutic effects and memory disturbances in treatment of endogenous depression with the Elther ES electroshock apparatus and Siemens Konvulsator III. J Nerv Ment Dis 137:268–276, 1963

Culver CM, Ferrell RB, Green RM: ECT and special problems of informed consent. Am J Psychiatry 137:586–591, 1980

Daniel WF, Crovitz HF: Acute memory impairment following electroconvulsive therapy, 2: effects of electrode placement. Acta Psychiatr Scand 67:57–68, 1983

Daniel WF, Crovitz HF: Disorientation during electroconvulsive therapy. Technical, theoretical, and neuropsychological issues. Ann NY Acad Sci 462:293–306, 1986

Davidson J, McLeod M, Law-Yone B, Linnoila M: A comparison of electroconvulsive therapy and combined phenelzine-amitriptyline in refractory depression. Arch Gen Psychiatry 35:639–642, 1978

Dec GW Jr, Stern TA, Welch C: The effects of electroconvulsive therapy on serial electrocardiograms and serum cardiac enzyme values: a prospective study of depressed hospitalized inpatients. JAMA 253:2525–2529, 1985

Decina P, Malitz S, Sackeim HA, Holzer J, Yudofsky S: Cardiac arrest during ECT modified by beta-adrenergic blockade. Am J Psychiatry 141:298–300, 1984

Decina P, Guthrie EB, Sackeim HA, Kahn D, Malitz S: Continuation ECT in the management of relapses of major affective episodes. Acta Psychiatr Scand 75:559–562, 1987

d'Elia G: Unilateral electroconvulsive therapy. Acta Psychiatr Scand [Suppl] 215:5–98, 1970

deQuardo JR, Tandon R: ECT in post-stroke major depression. Convulsive Therapy 4:221–224, 1988

Devanand DP, Sackeim HA: Seizure elicitation blocked by pretreatment with lidocaine. Convulsive Therapy 4:225–229, 1988

Devanand DP, Decina P, Sackeim HA, Prudic J: Status epilepticus during ECT in a patient receiving theophylline (letter). J Clin Psychopharmacol 8:153, 1988a

Devanand DP, Sackeim HA, Decina P, Prudic J: The development of mania and organic euphoria during ECT. J Clin Psychiatry 49:69–71, 1988b

Devanand D, Briscoe K, Sackeim H: Clinical features and predictors of postictal excitement. Convulsive Therapy 5:140–146, 1989

Devinsky O, Duchowny MS: Seizures after convulsive therapy: a retrospective case survey. Neurology 33:921–925, 1983

Dinwiddie SH, Drevetsw WC, Smith DR: Treatment of phencyclidine-associated psychosis with ECT. Convulsive Therapy 4:230–235, 1988

Dorn JB: Electroconvulsive therapy with fetal monitoring in a bipolar pregnant patient. Convulsive Therapy 1:217–221, 1985

Douglas CJ, Schwartz HI: ECT for depression caused by lupus cerebritis: a case report. Am J Psychiatry 139:1631–1632, 1982

Drop L, Welch C: Anesthesia for electroconvulsive therapy in patients with major cardiovascular risk factors. Convulsive Therapy 5:88–101, 1989

Dubois JC: Obsessions and mood: apropos of 43 cases of obsessive neurosis treated with antidepressive chemotherapy and electroshock. Ann Med Psychol (Paris) 142:141–151, 1984

Dubovsky SL: Using electroconvulsive therapy for patients with neurological disease. Hosp Community Psychiatry 37:819–825, 1986

Dudley WH Jr, Williams JG: Electroconvulsive therapy in delirium tremens. Compr Psychiatry 13:357–360, 1972

Dysken M, Evans HM, Chan CH, Davis JM: Improvement of depression and parkinsonism during ECT: a case study. Neuropsychobiology 2:81–86, 1976

el-Mallakh RS: Complications of concurrent lithium and electroconvulsive therapy: a review of clinical material and theoretical considerations. Biol Psychiatry 23:595–601, 1988

Fahy P, Imlah N, Harrington JA: A controlled comparison of electroconvulsive therapy, imipramine and thiopentone sleep in depression. Journal of Neuropsychiatry 4:310–314, 1963

Finestone DH, Weiner RD: Effects of ECT on diabetes mellitus: an attempt to account for conflicting data. Acta Psychiatr Scand 70:321–326, 1984

Fink M: Convulsive Therapy: Theory and Practice. New York, Raven Press, 1979

Fink M: Training in convulsive therapy (editorial). Convulsive Therapy 2:227–230, 1986

Fink M: ECT: a last resort treatment for resistant depression? in Treating Resistant Depression. Edited by Zohar J, Belmaker RH. New York, PMA Publishing, 1987a, pp 163–174

Fink M: Maintenance ECT and affective disorders. Convulsive Therapy 3:249–250, 1987b

Fink M: Convulsive therapy: a manual of practice, in American Psychiatric Press Review of Psychiatry, Vol 7. Edited by Frances AJ, Hales RE. Washington, DC, American Psychiatric Press, 1988, pp 482–497

Fink M: Reversible and irreversible dementia (editorial). Convulsive Therapy 5:123–125, 1989

Flor-Henry P: Electroconvulsive therapy and lateralized affective systems. Ann NY Acad Sci 462:389–397, 1986

Folstein M, Folstein S, McHugh P: "Mini-Mental State." J Psychiatric Res 12:189–198, 1975

Freeman CP, Kendell RE: Patients' experiences of and attitudes to electroconvulsive therapy. Ann NY Acad Sci 462:341–352, 1986

Freeman CP, Basson JV, Crighton A: Double-blind controlled trial of electroconvulsive therapy (E.C.T.) and simulated E.C.T. in depressive illness. Lancet 1:738–740, 1978

Freese KJ: Can patients safely undergo electroconvulsive therapy while receiving monoamine oxidase inhibitors? Convulsive Therapy 1:190–194, 1985

Fried D, Mann JJ: Electroconvulsive treatment of a patient with known intracranial tumor. Biol Psychiatry 23:176–180, 1988

Friedel RO: The combined use of neuroleptics and ECT in drug resistant schizophrenic patients. Psychopharmacol Bull 22:928–930, 1986

Gaines GY III, Rees DI: Electroconvulsive therapy and anesthetic considerations. Anesth Analg 65:1345–1356, 1986

Gaitz CM, Pokorny AD, Mills MJ: Death following electroconvulsive therapy. Arch Neurol Psychiatry 75:493–499, 1956

Gangadhar BN, Kapur RL, Kalyanasundaram S: Comparison of electroconvulsive therapy with imipramine in endogenous depression: a double blind study. Br J Psychiatry 141:367–371, 1982

Geretsegger C, Rochawanski E: Electroconvulsive therapy in acute life-threatening catatonia with associated cardiac and respiratory decompensation. Convulsive Therapy 3:291–295, 1987

Gerring JP, Shields HM: The identification and management of patients with a high risk for cardiac arrhythmias during modified ECT. J Clin Psychiatry 43:140–143, 1982

Greenan J, Dewar M, Jones C: Intravenous glycopyrrolate and atropine at the induction of anaethesia: a comparison. J R Soc Med 76:369–371, 1985

Greenberg LB, Anand A, Roque CT, Grinberg Y: Electroconvulsive therapy and cerebral venous angioma. Convulsive Therapy 2:197–202, 1986

Greenberg LB, Mofson R, Fink M: Prospective electroconvulsive therapy in a delusional depressed patient with a frontal meningioma: a case report. Br J Psychiatry 153:105–107, 1988

Greenblatt M, Grosser GH, Wechsler HA: Differential response of hospitalized depressed patients in somatic therapy. Am J Psychiatry 120:935–943, 1964

Gregory S, Shawcross CR, Gill D: The Nottingham ECT study: a double-blind comparison of bilateral, unilateral and simulated ECT in depressive illness. Br J Psychiatry 146:520–524, 1985

Group for the Advancement of Psychiatry: Shock Therapy. GAP Report No. 1, 1947

Group for the Advancement of Psychiatry: Revised Electro-Shock Therapy Report. GAP Report No. 15, 1950

Gruber RP: ECT for obsessive-compulsive symptoms (possible mechanisms of action). Diseases of the Nervous System 32:180–182, 1971

Grunhaus L, Dilsaver S, Greden JF, Carroll BJ: Depressive pseudo-dementia: a suggested diagnostic profile. Biol Psychiatry 18:215–225, 1983

Gujavarty K, Greenberg LB, Fink M: Electroconvulsive therapy and neuroleptic medication in therapy-resistant positive-symptom psychosis. Convulsive Therapy 3:111–120, 1987

Gutheil TG, Bursztajn H: Clinician's guidelines for assessing and presenting subtle forms of patient incompetence in legal settings. Am J Psychiatry 137:586–591, 1986

Guttmacher LB, Cretella H: Electroconvulsive therapy in one child and three adolescents. J Clin Psychiatry 49:20–23, 1988

Guze BH, Weinman B, Diamond RP: Use of ECT to treat bipolar depression in a mental retardate with cerebral palsy. Convulsive Therapy 3:60–64, 1987

Guze SB: The occurrence of psychiatric illness in systemic lupus erythematosus. Am J Psychiatry 123:1562–1570, 1967

Hafeiz HB: Psychiatric manifestations of enteric fever. Acta Psychiatr Scand 75:69–73, 1987

Hamilton M: Electroconvulsive therapy: indications and contraindications. Ann NY Acad Sci 462:5–11, 1986

Harris AJ: Harris Tests of Lateral Dominance. New York, Psychological Corp, 1958

Hermesh H, Shalev A, Weizman A, Aizenberg D: Neuroleptic malignant syndrome. Br J Psychiatry 149:384–385, 1986

Hermle L, Oepen G: Differential diagnosis of acute life threatening catatonia and malignant neuroleptic syndrome—a case report. Fortschr Neurol Psychiatr 54:189–195, 1986

Herzog A, Detre T: Psychotic reactions associated with childbirth. Diseases of the Nervous System 37:229–235, 1976

Heshe J, Roeder E: Electroconvulsive therapy in Denmark. Review of the technique, employment, indications and complications. Ugeskr Laeger 137:939–944, 1975

Hinkle PE, Coffey CE, Weiner RD, Cress M, Christison C: Use of caffeine to lengthen seizures in ECT. Am J Psychiatry 144:1143–1148, 1987

Holmberg G: The influence of oxygen administration on electrically induced convulsions in man. Acta Psychiatrica et Neurologica Scandinavica 28:365–386, 1953

Hood DD, Mecca RS: Failure to initiate electroconvulsive seizures in a patient pretreated with lidocaine. Anesthesiology 58:379–381, 1983

House A: Depression after stroke. Br Med J 294:76–78, 1987

Hsiao JK, Messenheimer JA, Evans DL: ECT and Neurological Disorders. Convulsive Therapy 3:121–136, 1987

Husum B, Vester-Andersen T, Buchmann G, Bolwig TG: Electroconvulsive therapy and intracranial aneurysm. Prevention of blood pressure elevation in a normotensive patient by hydralazine and propranolol. Anaesthesia 38:1205–1207, 1983

Hutchinson JT, Smedberg D: Treatment of depression: a comparative study of ECT and six drugs. Br J Psychiatry 109:536–538, 1963

Imlah NW, Ryan E, Harrington JA: The influence of antidepressant drugs on the response to electroconvulsive therapy and on subsequent relapse rates. Neuropsychopharmacology 4:438–442, 1965

Ingvar M: Cerebral blood flow and metabolic rate during seizures: relationship to epileptic brain damage. Ann NY Acad Sci 462:194–206, 1986

Janakiramaiah N, Channabasavanna SM, Murthy NS: ECT/chlorpromazine combination versus chlorpromazine alone in acutely schizophrenic patients. Acta Psychiatr Scand 66:464–470, 1982

Janicak PG, Easton M, Comaty JE, Dowd S, David JM: Efficacy of ECT in psychotic and nonpsychotic depression. Convulsive Therapy 5:314–320, 1989

Janike MA, Baer L, Minichiello WE: Somatic treatments for obsessive-compulsive disorders. Compr Psychiatry 28:250–263, 1987

Johnstone EC, Deakin JF, Lawler P, Frith CD, Stevens M, McPherson K, Crow TJ: The Northwick Park electroconvulsive therapy trial. Lancet 2:1317–1320, 1980

Kalinowsky LB, Hoch PH: Shock Treatments and Other Somatic Procedures in Psychiatry. New York, Grune & Stratton, 1946

Kalinowsky LB, Hoch PH: Somatic Treatments in Psychiatry. New York, Grune & Stratton, 1961

Kantor SJ, Glassman AH: Delusional depressions: natural history and response to treatment. Br J Psychiatry 131:351–360, 1977

Kay DW, Fahy T, Garside RF: A seven-month double-blind trial of amitriptyline and diazepam in ECT-treated depressed patients. Br J Psychiatry 117:667–671, 1970

Kellam AMP: The neuroleptic malignant syndrome. Br J Psychiatry 150:752–759, 1987

Keller MB, Lavori PW, Klerman GL, Andreasen NC, Endicott J, Coryell W, Fawcett J, Rice JP, Hirschfeld RM: Low levels and lack of predictors of somatotherapy and psychotherapy received by depressed patients. Arch Gen Psychiatry 43:458–466, 1986

Kellway B, Simpson K, Smith R, Halsall P: Effects of atropine and glycopyrrolate on cognitive function following anaesthesia and electroconvulsive therapy. Int Clin Psychopharmacol 1:296–302, 1986

Khanna S, Gangadhar BN, Sinha V, Rajendra PN, Channabasavanna SM: Electroconvulsive therapy in obsessive-compulsive disorder. Convulsive Therapy 4:314–320, 1988

Kiloh LG, Child JP, Latner G: A controlled trial of iproniazid in the treatment of endogenous depression. Journal of Mental Science 106:1139–1144, 1960

Kiloh LG, Smith JS, Johnson GF: Physical Treatments in Psychiatry. Melbourne, Australia, Blackwell Scientific, 1988

King PD: Phenelzine and ECT in the treatment of depression. Am J Psychiatry 116:64–68, 1959

Klein D, Gittelman R, Quitkin F, Rifkin A: Diagnosis and Drug Treatment of Psychiatric Disorders: Adults and Children. Baltimore, Williams and Wilkins, 1980

Knitter H: Experiences using electroconvulsive therapy in psychoses in childhood. Padiatr Grenzgeb 25:449–52, 1986

Kramer BA: Maintenance ECT: a survey of practice (1986). Convulsive Therapy 3:260–268, 1987

Kramp P, Bolwig TG: Electroconvulsive therapy in acute delirious states. Compr Psychiatry 22:368–371, 1981

Kristiansen ES: A comparison of treatment of endogenous depression with electroshock and with imipramine. Acta Psychiatr Scand 37:179–188, 1961

Kroessler D: Relative efficacy rates for therapies of delusional depression. Convulsive Therapy 1:173–182, 1985

Lambourn J, Gill D: A controlled comparison of simulated and real ECT. Br J Psychiatry 133:514–519, 1978

Langsley DG, Yager J: The definition of a psychiatrist: eight years later. Am J Psychiatry 145:469–475, 1988

Latey RH, Fahy TJ: ECT in the Republic of Ireland, 1982. Galway, Ireland, Galway University Press, 1985

Lebensohn ZM, Jenkins RB: Improvement of parkinsonism in depressed patients treated with ECT. Am J Psychiatry 132:283–285, 1975

Lerer B, Weiner RD, Belmaker RH: ECT: Basic Mechanisms. Washington, DC, American Psychiatric Press, 1986

Löo H, Galinowski A, Boccara I, Richard A: Value of maintenance electroshock therapy in recurrent depression: apropos of 4 cases. Encephale 14:39–41, 1988

Mac DS, Pardo MP: Systemic lupus erythematosus and catatonia: a case report. J Clin Psychiatry 44:155–156, 1983

Magni G, Fisman M, Helmes E: Clinical correlates of ECT-resistant depression in the elderly. J Clin Psychiatry 49:405–407, 1988

Mahler H, Co BT Jr, Dinwiddie S: Studies in involuntary civil commitment and involuntary electroconvulsive therapy. J Nerv Ment Dis 174:97–106, 1986

Maletzky BM: Seizure duration and clinical effect in electroconvulsive therapy. Compr Psychiatry 19:541–550, 1978

Maletzky B: Multiple-Monitored Electroconvulsive Therapy. Boca Raton, Fla, CRC Press, 1981

Malitz S, Sackeim, HA: Electroconvulsive Therapy: Clinical and Basic Research Issues. New York, New York Academy of Sciences, 1986

Maltbie AA, Wingfield MS, Volow MR, Weiner RD, Sullivan JL, Cavenar JO Jr: Electroconvulsive therapy in the presence of brain tumor: case reports and an evaluation of risk. J Nerv Ment Dis 168:400–405, 1980

Mann SC, Caroff SN, Bleier HR, Welz WK, Kling MA, Hayashida M: Lethal catatonia. Am J Psychiatry 143:1374–1381, 1986

Marco LA, Randels PM: Succinylcholine drug interactions during electroconvulsive therapy. Biol Psychiatry 14:433–445, 1979

Matzen TA, Martin RL, Watt TJ, Reilly DK: The use of maintenance ECT for relapsing depression. Jefferson Journal of Psychiatry 6:52–58, 1988

May PR: Treatment of Schizophrenia: A Comparative Study of Five Treatment Methods. New York, Science House, 1968

McAllister TW, Price TR: Severe depressive pseudodementia with and without dementia. Am J Psychiatry 139:626–629, 1982

McCabe MS: ECT in the treatment of mania: a controlled study. Am J Psychiatry 133:688–691, 1976

McCabe MS, Norris B: ECT versus chlorpromazine in mania. Biol Psychiatry 12:245–254, 1977

McDonald IM, Perkins M, Marjerrison G, Podilsky M: A controlled comparison of amitriptyline and electroconvulsive therapy in the treatment of depression. Am J Psychiatry 122:1427–1431, 1966

Medical Research Council: Clinical trial of the treatment of depressive illness. Br Med J 1:881–886, 1965

Meduna L: Die Konvulsionstherapie der Schizophrenie. Halle, Germany, Carl Marhold, 1937

Meisel A, Roth LH: Toward an informed discussion of informed consent. Ariz Law Rev 25:265–346, 1983

Mellman LA, Gorman JM: Successful treatment of obsessive-compulsive disorder with ECT. Am J Psychiatry 141:596–597, 1984

Miller AL, Faber RA, Hatch JP, Alexander HE: Factors affecting amnesia, seizure duration, and efficacy in ECT. Am J Psychiatry 142:692–696, 1985

Miller ME, Siris SG, Gabriel AN: Treatment delays in the course of electroconvulsive therapy. Hosp Community Psychiatry 37:825–827, 1986

Miller ME, Gabriel A, Herman G, Stern A, Shagong U, Kupersmith J: Atropine sulfate premedication and cardiac arrhythmia in electroconvulsive therapy. Convulsive Therapy 3:10–17, 1987

Mills MJ, Avery D: The legal regulation of electroconvulsive therapy, in Mood Disorders: The World's Major Public Health Problem. Edited by Ayd FJ. Baltimore, Frank Ayd Communications, 1978, pp 154–183

Milstein V, Small JG: Problems with lithium combined with ECT (letter). Am J Psychiatry 145:1178, 1988

Milstein V, Small JG, Small IF, Green GE: Does electroconvulsive therapy prevent suicide? Convulsive Therapy 2:3–6, 1986

Milstein V, Small JG, Klapper MH, Small IF, Kellams JJ: Uni- versus bilateral ECT in the treatment of mania. Convulsive Therapy 3:1–9, 1987

Minter RE, Mandel MR: The treatment of psychotic major depressive disorder with drugs and electroconvulsive therapy. J Nerv Ment Dis 167:726–733, 1979

Mukherjee S, Sackeim HA, Lee C, et al: ECT in treatment resistant mania, in Biological Psychiatry 1985. Edited by Shagass C, Josiassen RC, Bridger WH, et al. New York, Elsevier, 1986, pp 732–734

Mukherjee S, Sackeim HA, Lee C: Unilateral ECT in the treatment of manic episodes. Convulsive Therapy 4:74–80, 1988

Murray GB, Shea V, Conn DK: Electroconvulsive therapy for poststroke depression. J Clin Psychiatry 47:258–260, 1986

Nelson JP, Benjamin L: Efficacy and safety of combined ECT and tricyclic antidepressant therapy in the treatment of depressed geriatric patients. Convulsive Therapy 5:321–329, 1989

Nettlebladt P: Factors influencing number of treatments and seizure duration in ECT: drug treatment, social class. Convulsive Therapy 4:160–168, 1988

Nilsen SM, Willis KW, Pettinati HM: Initial impression of two new brief-pulse electroconvulsive therapy machines. Convulsive Therapy 2:43–54, 1986

Norris AS, Clancy J: Hospitalized depressions: drugs or electrotherapy. Arch Gen Psychiatry 5:276–279, 1961

Nurnberg HG, Prudic J: Guidelines for treatment of psychosis during pregnancy. Hosp Community Psychiatry 35:67–71, 1984

O'Shea B, Lynch T, Falvey J, O'Mahoney G: Electroconvulsive therapy and cognitive improvement in a very elderly depressed patient. Br J Psychiatry 150:255–257, 1987

O'Toole JK, Dyck G: Report of psychogenic fever in catatonia responding to electroconvulsive therapy. Diseases of the Nervous System 38:852–853, 1977

Oates MR: The treatment of psychiatric disorders in pregnancy and the puerperium. Clin Obstet Gynecol 13:385–395, 1986

Ontario Ministry of Health: Report of the Electro-Convulsive Review Committee. Toronto, Ontario Ministry of Health, 1985

Ottosson J-O: Experimental studies of the mode of action of electroconvulsive therapy. Acta Psychiatr Scand [Suppl] 145:1–141, 1960

Pankratz WJ: Electroconvulsive therapy: the position of the Canadian Psychiatric Association. Can J Psychiatry 25:509–514, 1980

Parry J: Legal parameters of informed consent for ECT administered to mentally disabled persons. Psychopharmacol Bull 22:490–494, 1986

Paul SM, Extein I, Calil HM, Potter WZ, Chodoff P, Goodwin FK: Use of ECT with treatment-resistant depressed patients at the National Institute of Mental Health. Am J Psychiatry 138:486–489, 1981

Pearlman CA: Neuroleptic malignant syndrome: a review of the literature. J Clin Psychopharmacol 6:257–273, 1986

Perris C, d'Elia G: A study of bipolar (manic-depressive) and unipolar recurrent depressive psychoses, IX: therapy and prognosis. Acta Psychiatr Scand [Suppl] 194:153–171, 1966

Peters SG, Wochos DN, Peterson GC: Status epilepticus as a complication of concurrent electroconvulsive and theophylline therapy. Mayo Clin Proc 59:568–570, 1984

Pettinati HM, Mathisen KS, Rosenberg J, Lynch JF: Meta-analytical approach to reconciling discrepancies in efficacy between bilateral and unilateral electroconvulsive therapy. Convulsive Therapy 2:7–17, 1986

Pettinati HM, Willis KW, Nilsen SM, Robin SE: Benzodiazepines reduce ECT's therapeutic effect, in Abstracts of the 140th Annual Meeting of the American Psychiatric Association, May 1987

Pippard J, Ellam L: Electroconvulsive Treatment in Great Britain. London, Gaskell, 1981

Pitts FN Jr: Medical physiology of ECT, in Electroconvulsive Therapy: Biological Foundations and Clinical Applications. Edited by Abrams R, Essman W. New York, Spectrum Publications, 1982, pp 57–90

Pitts FN Jr, Patterson CW: Electroconvulsive therapy for iatrogenic hypothalamic-hypopituitarism (CRF-ACTH type). Am J Psychiatry 136:1074–1077, 1979

Pomeranze J, Karliner W, Triebel WA, King EJ: Electroshock therapy in presence of serious organic disease. Depression and aortic aneurysm. Geriatrics 23:122–124, 1968

Pope HG Jr, Lipinski JF, Cohen BM, Axelrod DT: "Schizoaffective disorder": an invalid diagnosis? A comparison of schizoaffective disorder, schizophrenia, and affective disorder. Am J Psychiatry 137:921–927, 1980

Pope HG, Keck PE, McElroy SL: Frequency and presentation of neuroleptic malignant syndrome in a large psychiatric hospital. Am J Psychiatry 143:1227–1233, 1986

Pratt RT, Warrington EK, Halliday AM: Unilateral ECT as a test for cerebral dominance, with a strategy for treating left-handers. Br J Psychiatry 119:79–83, 1971

Price TR, McAllister TW: Response of depressed patients to sequential unilateral nondominant brief-pulse and bilateral sinusoidal ECT. J Clin Psychiatry 47:182–186, 1986

Protheroe C: Puerperal psychoses: a long-term study, 1927–1961. Br J Psychiatry 115:9–30, 1969

Prudic J, Sackeim HA, Decina P, Hopkins N, Ross FR, Malitz S: Acute effects of ECT on cardiovascular functioning: relations to patient and treatment variables. Acta Psychiatr Scand 75:344–351, 1987

Prudic J, Sackeim H, Devanand D: Medication resistance and clinical response to electroconvulsive therapy. Psychiatry Res (in press)

Quitkin FM, Rabkin JG, Ross D, McGrath PJ: Duration of antidepressant drug treatment: what is an adequate trial? Arch Gen Psychiatry 41:238–245, 1984

Räsänen J, Martin DJ, Downs JB, Hodges MR: Oxygen supplementation during electroconvulsive therapy. Br J Anaesth 61:593–597, 1988

Raskin DE: A survey of electroconvulsive therapy: use and training in university hospitals in 1984 (letter). Convulsive Therapy 2:293–299, 1986

Regestein QR, Reich P: Electroconvulsive therapy in patients at high risk for physical complications. Convulsive Therapy 1:101–114, 1985

Remick RA, Jewesson P, Ford RWJ: MAO inhibitors in general anesthesia: a re-evaluation. Convulsive Therapy 3:196–203, 1987

Repke JT, Berger NG: Electroconvulsive therapy in pregnancy. Obstet Gynecol 63:39S–41S, 1984

Rich C, Woodruff R, Cadoret R, Craig A, Pitts F: Electrotherapy: the effects of atropine on EKG. Diseases of the Nervous System 30:622–626, 1969

Ries RK, Wilson L, Bokan JA, Chiles JA: ECT in medication resistant schizoaffective disorder. Compr Psychiatry 22:167–173, 1981

Robin AA, Harris JA: A controlled trial of imipramine and electroplexy. Journal of Mental Science 106:217–219, 1962

Robin A, de Tissera S: A double-blind controlled comparison of the therapeutic effects of low and high energy electroconvulsive therapies. Br J Psychiatry 141:357–366, 1982

Robin A, Binnie CD, Copas JB: Electrophysiological and hormonal responses to three types of electroconvulsive therapy. Br J Psychiatry 147:707–712, 1985

Robinson GE, Stewart DE: Postpartum psychiatric disorders. Can Med Assoc J 134:31–37, 1986

Rodin G, Voshart K: Depression in the medically ill: an overview. Am J Psychiatry 143:696–705, 1986

Rosen AM, Mukherjee S, Shinbach K: The efficacy of ECT in phencyclidine-induced psychosis. J Clin Psychiatry 45:220–222, 1984

Roth LH: Data on informed consent for ECT. Psychopharmacol Bull 22:494–495, 1986

Roth LH, Meisel A, Lidz CW: Tests of competency to consent for treatment. Am J Psychiatry 134:279–284, 1977

Roth LH, Lidz CW, Meisel A, Soloff PH, Kaufman K, Spiker DG, Foster FG: Competency to decide about treatment and research: an overview of some empirical data. Int J Law Psychiatry 5:29–50, 1982

Roth SD, Mukherjee SS: Electroconvulsive therapy in a patient with mania, parkinsonism, and tardive dyskinesia. Convulsive Therapy 4:92–97, 1988

Royal College of Nursing: RCN nursing guidelines for ECT. Convulsive Therapy 3:158–160, 1987

Royal College of Psychiatrists: Memorandum on the use of ECT. Br J Psychiatry 131:261–272, 1977

Royal College of Psychiatrists: The practical administration of electroconvulsive therapy (ECT). London, Gaskell, 1989

Roy-Byrne P, Gerner RH: Legal restrictions on the use of ECT in California: clinical impact on the incompetent patient. J Clin Psychiatry 42:300–303, 1981

Roy-Byrne P, Gerner RH, Lisoton EH, Robertson AG: ECT for acute mania: a forgotten treatment modality? Journal of Psychiatric Treatment and Evaluation 3:83–86, 1981

Rudorfer MV, Linnoila M, Potter WZ: Combined lithium and electroconvulsive therapy: pharmacokinetic and pharmacodynamic interactions. Convulsive Therapy 3:40–45, 1987

Russell EW: Renorming Russell's Version of the Wechsler Memory Scale. J Clin Exp Neuropsychol 10:235–249, 1988

Sackeim HA, Steif BL: The neuropsychology of depression and mania, in Depression and Mania. Edited by Georgotas A, Cancro R. New York, Elsevier, 1988, pp 265–289

Sackeim HA, Greenberg MS, Weiman AL, Gur RC, Hungerbuhler JP, Geschwind N: Hemispheric asymmetry in the expression of positive and negative emotions: neurologic evidence. Arch Neurol 39:210–218, 1982

Sackeim HA, Decina P, Prohovnik I, Malitz S, Resor S: Anticonvulsant and antidepressant properties of ECT: a proposed mechanism of action. Biol Psychiatry 18:1301–1310, 1983

Sackeim HA, Portnoy S, Neeley P, Steif BL, Decina P, Malitz S: Cognitive consequences of low-dosage electroconvulsive therapy. Ann NY Acad Sci 462:326–340, 1986a

Sackeim HA, Decina P, Prohovnik I, Portnoy S, Kanzler M, Malitz S: Dosage, seizure threshold, and the antidepressant efficacy of electroconvulsive therapy. Ann NY Acad Sci 462:398–410, 1986b

Sackeim H, Ross F, Hopkins N, Calev L, Devanand D: Subjective side effects acutely following ECT: associations with treatment modality and clinical response. Convulsive Therapy 3:100–110, 1987a

Sackeim HA, Decina P, Kanzler M, Kerr B, Malitz S: Effects of electrode placement on the efficacy of titrated, low-dose ECT. Am J Psychiatry 144:1449–1455, 1987b

Sackeim H, Decina P, Prohovnik I, Malitz S: Seizure threshold in electroconvulsive therapy: effects of sex, age, electrode placement, and number of treatments. Arch Gen Psychiatry 44:355–360, 1987c

Sackeim HA, Decina P, Portnoy S, Neeley P, Malitz S: Studies of dosage, seizure threshold, and seizure duration in ECT. Biol Psychiatry 22:249–268, 1987d

Sackeim HA, Prudic J, Devanand DP: Treatment of medication-resistant depression with electroconvulsive therapy, in American Psychiatric Press Review of Psychiatry, Vol 9. Edited by Tasman A, Goldfinger SM, Kaufmann CA. Washington, DC, American Psychiatric Press, 1990, pp 91–115

Sackeim H, Prudic J, Devanand D, Decina P, Kerr B, Malitz S: The impact of medication resistance and continuation pharmacotherapy on relapse following response to electroconvulsive therapy in major depression. J Clin Psychopharmacol (in press)

Salzman C: ECT and ethical psychiatry. Am J Psychiatry 134:1006–1009, 1977

Salzman C: The use of ECT in the treatment of schizophrenia. Am J Psychiatry 137:1032–1041, 1980

Sargant W, Slater E: An Introduction to Physical Methods of Treatment in Psychiatry, 3rd ed. Baltimore, Williams & Wilkins, 1954

Sargant W, Slater E: An Introduction to Physical Methods of Treatment in Psychiatry, 5th ed. Baltimore, Williams & Wilkins, 1963

Schnur D, Mukherjee S, Silver J, Degreef G, Lee C: ECT in the treatment of episodic aggressive dyscontrol in psychotic patients. Convulsive Therapy 5:353–361, 1989

Scott AIF, Riddle W: Status epilepticus after electroconvulsive therapy. Br J Psychiatry 155:119–121, 1989

Seager CR, Bird RL: Imipramine with electrical treatment in depression—a controlled trial. Journal of Mental Science 108:704–707, 1962

Selvin BL: Electroconvulsive therapy—1987. Anesthesiology 67:367–385, 1987

Shapira B, Zohar J, Newman M, Drexler H, Belmaker RH: Potentiation of seizure length and clinical response to electroconvulsive therapy by caffeine pretreatment: a case report. Convulsive Therapy 1:58–60, 1985

Shapira B, Lerer B, Gilboa D, Drexler H, Kugelmass S, Calev A: Facilitation of ECT by caffeine pretreatment. Am J Psychiatry 144:1199–1202, 1987

Shugar G, Hoffman BF, Johnston JD: Electroconvulsive therapy for schizophrenia in Ontario: a report on therapeutic polymorphism. Compr Psychiatry 25:509–520, 1984

Siesjö BK, Ingvar M, Wieloch T: Cellular and molecular events underlying epileptic brain damage. Ann NY Acad Sci 462:207–223, 1986

Simon JS, Evans D: Pheochromocytoma, depression and electroconvulsive therapy. Convulsive Therapy 2:296–298, 1986

Small JG: Efficacy of electroconvulsive therapy in schizophrenia, mania, and other disorders, I: Schizophrenia. II: Mania and other disorders. Convulsive Therapy 1:263–270, 271–276, 1985

Small JG, Kellams JJ, Milstein V, Small IF: Complications with electroconvulsive treatment combined with lithium. Biol Psychiatry 15:103–112, 1980

Small JG, Milstein V, Small IF, Sharpley PH: Does ECT produce kindling? Biol Psychiatry 16:773–778, 1981

Small JG, Milstein V, Klapper MH, Kellams JJ, Small IF: ECT combined with neuroleptics in the treatment of schizophrenia. Psychopharmacol Bull 18:34–35, 1982

Small JG, Klapper MH, Kellams JJ, Miller MJ, Milstein V, Sharpley PH, Small IF: Electroconvulsive treatment compared with lithium in the management of manic states. Arch Gen Psychiatry 45:727–732, 1988

Smith K, Surphlis W, Gynther M, Shimkunas AM: ECT-chlorpromazine and chlorpromazine compared in the treatment of schizophrenia. J Nerv Ment Dis 144:284–292, 1967

Snaith RP: How much ECT does the depressed patient need? in Electroconvulsive Therapy: an Appraisal. Edited by Palmer RL. New York, Oxford University Press, 1981, pp 61–64

Spiker D, Stein J, Rich CL: Delusional depression and electroconvulsive therapy: one year later. Convulsive Therapy 1:167–172, 1985

Squire LR: Memory functions as affected by electroconvulsive therapy. Ann NY Acad Sci 462:307–314, 1986

Squire LR, Wetzel CD, Slater PC: Memory complaint after electroconvulsive therapy: assessment with a new self-rating instrument. Biol Psychiatry 14:791–801, 1979

Standish-Barry HM, Deacon V, Snaith RP: The relationship of concurrent benzodiazepine administration to seizure duration in ECT. Acta Psychiatr Scand 71:269–271, 1985

Stanley WJ, Fleming H: A clinical comparison of phenelzine and electro-convulsive therapy in the treatment of depressive illness. Journal of Mental Science 108:708–710, 1962

Steif BL, Sackeim HA, Portnoy S, Decina P, Malitz S: Effects of depression and ECT on anterograde memory. Biol Psychiatry 21:921–930, 1986

Stephens SM, Pettinati HM, Willis KW, Bedient L, Greenberg RM, Zomorodi A: Clinical review of Medcraft Corporations's new brief-pulse ECT device. Convulsive Therapy 6:42–53, 1990

Sternberg DE, Jarvik ME: Memory function in depression: improvement with antidepressant medication. Arch Gen Psychiatry 33:219–224, 1976

Strain JJ, Bidder TG: Transient cerebral complication associated with multiple monitored electroconvulsive therapy. Diseases of the Nervous System 32:95–100, 1971

Strömgren LS: Is bilateral ECT ever indicated? Acta Psychiatr Scand 69:484–490, 1984

Strömgren LS, Dahl J, Fjeldborg N, Thomsen A: Factors influencing seizure duration and number of seizures applied in unilateral electroconvulsive therapy: anaesthetics and benzodiazepines. Acta Psychiatr Scand 62:158–165, 1980

Swartz C, Saheba N: Comparison of atropine with glycopyrrolate for use in ECT. Convulsive Therapy 5:56–60, 1989

Tancer ME, Pedersen CA, Evans DL: ECT and anticoagulation. Convulsive Therapy 3:222–227, 1987

Taub S: Electroconvulsive therapy, malpractice, and informed consent. Journal of Psychiatry and Law 15:7–54, 1987

Taylor JR, Tompkins R, Demers R, Anderson D: Electroconvulsive therapy and memory dysfunction: is there evidence for prolonged defects? Biol Psychiatry 17:1169–1193, 1982

Taylor MA: Indications for ECT, in Electroconvulsive Therapy: Biological Foundations and Clinical Applications. Edited by Abrams R, Essman W. New York, Spectrum Publications, 1982, pp 7–40

Taylor MA, Abrams R: Catatonia: prevalence and importance in the manic phase of manic-depressive illness. Arch Gen Psychiatry 34:1223–1225, 1977

Taylor P, Fleminger JJ: ECT for schizophrenia. Lancet 1:1380–1382, 1980

Tenenbaum J: ECT regulation reconsidered. Medical Disability Law Reporter 7:148–159, 211, 1983

Thomas J, Reddy B: The treatment of mania: a retrospective evaluation of the effects of ECT, chlorpromazine, and lithium. J Affective Disord 4:85–92, 1982

Thornton JE, Mulsant BH, Reynolds CF: A descriptive study of maintenance electroconvulsive therapy (M-ECT) in geriatrics. Abstracts, Society of Biological Psychiatry, May 1988

Tsuang MT, Dempsey GM, Fleming JA: Can ECT prevent premature death and suicide in "schizoaffective" patients? J Affective Disord 1:167–171, 1979

Viby-Mogensen J, Hanel H: Prolonged apnea after suxamethonium. Acta Anaesth Scand 22:371–380, 1978

Walter-Ryan WG: ECT regulation and the two-tiered care system. Am J Psychiatry 142:661–662, 1985

Ward C, Stern GM, Pratt RT, McKenna P: Electroconvulsive therapy in Parkinsonian patients with the "on-off" syndrome. J Neural Transm 49:133–135, 1980

Warneke L: A case of manic-depressive illness in childhood. Canadian Psychiatric Association Journal 20:195–200, 1975

Weeks D, Freeman CP, Kendell RE: ECT, III: enduring cognitive deficits? Br J Psychiatry 137:26–37, 1980

Weiner RD: ECT and seizure threshold: effects of stimulus wave form and electrode placement. Biol Psychiatry 15:225–241, 1980

Weiner RD: The role of stimulus waveform and therapeutic and adverse effects of ECT. Psychopharmacol Bull 18:71–72, 1982

Weiner RD: Does electroconvulsive therapy cause brain damage? The Behavioral and Brain Sciences 7:1–54, 1984

Weiner RD, Coffey CE: Use of electroconvulsive therapy in patients with severe medical illness, in Treatment of Psychiatric Disorders in Medical-Surgical Patients. Edited by Stoudemire A, Fogel B. New York, Grune & Stratton, 1987, pp 113–134

Weiner RD, Coffey CE: Indications for use of electroconvulsive therapy, in American Psychiatric Press Review of Psychiatry, Vol 7. Edited by Frances AJ, Hales RE. Washington, DC, American Psychiatric Press, 1988, pp 458–481

Weiner RD, Whanger AD, Erwin CW, Wilson WP: Prolonged confusional state and EEG seizure activity following concurrent ECT and lithium use. Am J Psychiatry 137:1452–1453, 1980

Weiner RD, Rogers HJ, Davidson JR, Kahn EM: Effects of electroconvulsive therapy upon brain electrical activity. Ann NY Acad Sci 462:270–281, 1986a

Weiner RD, Rogers HJ, Davidson JR, Squire LR: Effects of stimulus parameters on cognitive side effects. Ann NY Acad Sci 462:315–325, 1986b

Welch C, Drop L: Cardivascular effects of ECT. Convulsive Therapy 5:35–43, 1989

Wells DG, Bjorkstein AR: Monoamine oxidase inhibitors revisited. Can J Anaesth 36:64–74, 1989

West ED: Electric convulsion therapy in depression: a double-blind controlled trial. Br Med J [Clin Res] 282:355–357, 1981

Wettstein RM, Roth LH: The psychiatrist as legal guardian. Am J Psychiatry 145:600–604, 1988

Wilson IC, Vernon JT, Guin T, Sandifer MG: A controlled study of treatments of depression. Journal of Neuropsychiatry 4:331–337, 1963

Winslade WJ: Electroconvulsive therapy: legal considerations and ethical concerns, in American Psychiatric Press Review of Psychiatry, Vol 7. Edited by Frances AJ, Hales RE. Washington, DC, American Psychiatric Press, pp 513–525, 1988

Winslade WJ, Liston EH, Ross JW, Weber KD: Medical, judicial, and statutory regulation of ECT in the United States. Am J Psychiatry 141:1349–1355, 1984

Wisner KL, Perel JM: Pharmacologic agents and electroconvulsive therapy during pregnancy and puerperium, in Psychiatric Consultation in Childbirth Settings: Parent and Child-Oriented Approaches. Edited by Cohen RL. New York, Plenum, 1988, pp 165–206

Wyant GM, MacDonald WB: The role of atropine in electroconvulsive therapy. Anaesth Intensive Care 8:445–450, 1980

Yager J, Borus JF, Robinowitz CB, Shore JH: Developing minimal national standards for clinical experience in psychiatric training. Am J Psychiatry 145:1409–1413, 1988

Zimmerman M, Coryell W, Pfohl B: The treatment validity of DSM-III melancholic subtyping. Psychiatry Res 16:37–43, 1985

Zorumski CF, Rutherford JL, Burke WJ, Reich T: ECT in primary and secondary depression. J Clin Psychiatry 47:298–300, 1986

Appendices

Appendix A

Individuals and Groups
Providing Input to the
Guidelines Development Process

To ensure that these guidelines were as accurate and comprehensive as possible, the APA Task Force on Electroconvulsive Therapy solicited and encouraged input on them from relevant groups both inside and outside of the American Psychiatric Association. While the document was in draft form, it was distributed to approximately 90 individuals and groups. Among these were academic experts and practitioners in relevant areas of psychiatry, anesthesiology, cardiology, nursing, and psychology.

Device manufacturers were given the opportunity to comment, as were regulatory organizations such as the Joint Commission on Accreditation of Health Care Organizations, the Food and Drug Administration, and governmental agencies such as the National Institute of Mental Health and the Veterans Administration. In addition, professional and scientific societies with an interest in ECT were asked to provide formal comments. Finally, major lay organizations representing the consumer and their families were also provided with the opportunity to review and comment on the guidelines. An additional opportunity was provided to those wishing to meet with the Task Force at a public meeting held at the American Psychiatric Association on January 12, 1989.

Within the APA component structure, the guidelines were shared with representatives focusing on problems of children, aging, law, governmental relations, public affairs, and education. In addition, the APA guidelines were made available to members of the Assembly of District Branches, and were reviewed in toto by members of the Committee on Research on Psychiatric Treatments, the Council on Research, the Joint Reference Committee, and finally by members of the Board of Trustees.

Below is a listing of organizations followed by a listing of individual experts who actually provided input into this document. Other individuals and groups were provided with the opportunity to comment but did not.

Representatives of the following organizations provided input into these guidelines

- Accreditation Council for Graduate Medical Education
- American Academy of Clinical Psychiatrists
- American Academy of Psychiatry and Law
- American Association of Chairmen of Departments of Psychiatry
- American Association of Directors of Psychiatric Residency Training
- American Association of General Hospital Psychiatrists
- American Hospital Association
- American Nurses Association
- American Psychological Association
- American Society of Anesthesiologists
- Association for Convulsive Therapy
- Association of Directors of Medical Student Education in Psychiatry
- Canadian Psychiatric Association
- Food and Drug Administration
- Joint Commission of Accreditation of Health Care Organizations
- MECTA Corporation
- National Alliance for the Mentally Ill
- National Association of Private Psychiatric Hospitals
- National Association of State Mental Health Program Directors
- National Depressive and Manic Depressive Association
- National Institute of Mental Health
- Royal College of Psychiatrists
- Somatics, Inc.
- Veterans Administration

**The following individuals provided comments
on the draft of the ECT Task Force Report:**

Richard Abrams, M.D
North Chicago, IL

James T. Barter, M.D.
Chicago, IL

T. George Bidder, M.D.
Sepulveda, CA

Joe Bona, M.D.
Durham, NC

J. C. N. Brown, M.D.
Iowa City, IA

Richard P. Brown, M.D.
New York, NY

Robert A. Burt
New Haven, CT

James S. Cheatham, M.D.
Atlanta, GA

Fred Cobb, M.D.
Durham, NC

C. Edward Coffey, M.D.
Durham, NC

Irvin Cohen, M.D.
Houston, TX

Jonathan O. Cole, M.D.
Brookline, MA

Raymond Crowe, M.D.
Iowa City, IA

Robert Dealy, M.D.
Pittsburgh, PA

Charles P. Deminico, M.D.
Tampa, FL

D. P. Devanand, M.D.
New York, NY

George Dyck, M.D.
Newton, KS

Norman Endler, Ph.D.
Toronto, Ontario, Canada

Ray Faber, M.D.
San Antonio, TX

Fred H. Frankel, M.D.
Boston, MA

Chris Freeman, M.B., Ch.B.,
M.R.C.Psych.
Edinburgh, Scotland

Michael Gluck, Sc.D.
Rockville, MD

Joel A. Griffith, M.D.
Indianapolis, IN

Edward Hanin, M.D.
Harrison, NY

Donald P. Hay, M.D.
Milwaukee, WI

Ms. Artie Houston
Fort Worth, TX

Barry Alan Kramer, M.D.
Los Angeles, CA

William Kammerer, M.D.
Bethesda, MD

David Kupfer, M.D.
Pittsburgh, PA

Zigmond Lebensohn, M.D.
Washington, DC

Stuart Levy, D.O.
Philadelphia, PA

Edward Liston, M.D.
Los Angeles, CA

Patrick Loren, M.D.
Washington, DC

Barry Maletsky, M.D.
Portland, OR

Sidney Malitz, M.D.
New York, NY

J. John Mann, M.D.
Pittsburgh, PA

Barry A. Martin, M.D.,
F.R.C.P. (C)
Montreal, Quebec, Canada

Myrene McAninch, Ph.D.
Chicago, IL

David L. McCann, M.D.
Holladay, Utah

Douglas McNair, Ph.D.
Boston, MA

Charles Miles, M.D.
Salt Lake City, UT

Victor Milstein, Ph.D.
Indianapolis, IN

Eric Moffet, M.D.
Durham, NC

Frank Moscarillo, M.D.
Washington, DC

Sukdeb Mukerjee, M.D.
New York, NY

Robin Nicol
Portland, OR

Joseph N. Onek, J.D.
Washington, DC

Chester Pearlman, M.D.
Brookline, MA

Barry Perlman, M.D.
Yonkers, NY

Glen N. Peterson, M.D.
Oakland, CA

Trevor Price, M.D.
Pittsburgh, PA

Robert Prien, Ph.D.
Rockville, MD

Joan Prudic, M.D.
New York, NY

John Racy, M.D.
Tucson, AZ

Lewis T. Ray, M.D.
San Francisco, CA

Robert Rose, M.D.
Minneapolis, MN

Loren H. Roth, M.D.
Pittsburgh, PA

Michael Schlesser, M.D.
Dallas, TX

Beatrice Selvin, M.D.
Crownsville, MD

James Shore, M.D.
Denver, CO

Karen Sibert, M.D.
Durham, NC

Larry B. Silver, M.D.
Potomac, MD

Joyce Small, M.D.
Indianapolis, IN

Philip J. Smeraski, M.D.
Greensville, NC

Gail Stuart, Ph.D., R.N.
Charleston, SC

Conrad Swartz, M.D., Ph.D.
Lake Bluff, IL

James M. Trench, M.D.
New London, CT

Charles A. Welch, M.D.
Boston, MA

Robert M. Wettstein, M.D.
Baltimore, MD

Sherwyn Woods, M.D., Ph.D.
Los Angeles, CA

Howard V. Zonana, M.D.
New Haven, CT

Appendix B

Examples of Consent Forms and Patient Information Sheet for an ECT Course

[Name of Facility Here]

ECT Consent Form

Name of Attending Physician: _____

Name of Patient: _____

    My doctor has recommended that I receive treatment with Electroconvulsive Therapy (ECT). The nature of this treatment, including the risks and benefits that I may experience, have been fully described to me and I give my consent to be treated with ECT.

    I will receive ECT to treat my psychiatric condition. I understand that there may be other alternative treatments for my condition which may include medications and psychotherapy. Whether ECT or an alternative treatment is most appropriate for me depends on my prior experience with these treatments, the nature of my psychiatric condition, and other considerations. Why ECT has been recommended for my specific case has been explained to me.

    ECT involves a series of treatments. To receive each treatment I will be brought to a specially equipped room in this facility. The treatments are usually given in the morning, before breakfast. Because the treatments involve general anesthesia, I will have had nothing to drink or eat for at least six hours before each treatment. When I come to the treatment room, an injection will be made in my vein so that I can be given medications. I will be given an anesthetic drug that will quickly put me to sleep. I will be given a second drug that will relax my muscles. Because I will be asleep, I will not experience pain or discomfort during the procedure. I will not feel the electrical current, and when I wake up I will have no memory of the treatment.

To prepare for the treatments, monitoring sensors will be placed on my head and other parts of my body. A blood pressure cuff will be placed on one of my limbs. This is done to monitor my brain waves, my heart, and my blood pressure. These recordings involve no pain or discomfort. After I am asleep, a small, carefully controlled amount of electricity will be passed between two electrodes that have been placed on my head. Depending on where the electrodes are placed, I may receive either bilateral ECT or unilateral ECT. In bilateral ECT, one electrode is placed on the left side of the head, the other on the right side. In unilateral ECT, both electrodes are placed on the same side of the head, usually on the right side. When the current is passed, a generalized seizure is produced in the brain. Because I will have been given a medication to relax my muscles, muscular contractions in my body that would ordinarily accompany a seizure will be considerably softened. The seizure will last for approximately one minute. Within a few minutes, the anesthetic drug will wear off and I will awaken. During the procedure my heart rate, blood pressure, and other functions will be monitored. I will be given oxygen to breathe. After waking up from the anesthesia, I will be brought to a recovery room, where I will be observed until it is time to leave the ECT area. The number of treatments that I receive cannot be predicted ahead of time. The number of treatments will depend on my psychiatric condition, how quickly I respond to the treatment, and the medical judgment of my psychiatrist. Typically, six to twelve treatments are given. However, some patients respond slowly and more treatments may be required. Treatments are usually given three times a week, but the frequency of treatment may also vary depending on my needs.

The potential benefit of ECT for me is that it may lead to improvement in my psychiatric condition. ECT has been shown to be a highly effective treatment for a number of conditions. However, not all patients respond equally well. As with all forms of medical treatment, some patients recover quickly; others recover only to relapse again and require further treatment, while still others fail to respond at all.

Like other medical procedures, ECT involves some risks. When I awaken after each treatment, I may experience confusion. The confusion usually goes away within an hour. Shortly after the treatment, I may have a headache, muscle soreness, or nausea. These side effects usually respond to simple treatment. More serious medical complications with ECT are rare. With modern ECT techniques, dislocations or bone fracture, and dental complications very rarely occur. As with any general anesthetic procedure, there is a remote possibility of death. It is estimated that fatality associated with ECT occurs approximately one per 10,000 patients treated. While also rare, the most common medical complications with ECT are irregularities in heart rate and rhythm.

To reduce the risk of medical complications, I will receive a careful medical evaluation prior to starting ECT. However, in spite of precautions there is a small chance that I will experience a medical complication. Should this occur, I understand that medical care and treatment will be instituted immediately and that facilities to handle emergencies are available. I understand, however, that neither the institution nor the treating physicians are required to provide long-term medical treatment. I shall be responsible for the cost of such treatment whether personally or through medical insurance or other medical coverage. I understand that no compensation will be paid for lost wages or other consequential damages.

A common side effect of ECT is poor memory functioning. The degree of disruption of memory is likely to be related to the number of treatments given and their type. A smaller number of treatments is likely to produce less memory impairment than a larger number of treatments. Right unilateral ECT (electrodes on the right-side) is likely to produce milder and shorter-lived memory impairment than that following bilateral ECT (one electrode on each side of the head). The memory difficulties with ECT have a characteristic pattern. Shortly following a treatment, the problems with memory are most pronounced. As time from treatment increases, memory functioning improves. Shortly after the course of ECT, I may experience difficulties remembering events that happened before and while I received ECT. This spottiness in memory for past events may extend back to several months before I received ECT, and in rare instances, to one or two years. Many of these memories will return during the first several months following the ECT course. However, I may be left with some permanent gaps in memory, particularly for events that occurred close in time to the ECT course. In addition, for a short period following ECT, I may experience difficulty in learning and remembering new information. This difficulty in forming new memories should be temporary and will most likely subside within several weeks following the ECT course.

Individuals vary considerably in the extent to which they experience confusion and memory problems during and shortly following treatment with ECT. However, in part because psychiatric conditions themselves produce impairments in learning and memory, many patients actually report that their learning and memory functioning is improved after ECT compared to their functioning prior to the treatment course. A small minority of patients, perhaps 1 in 200, report severe problems in memory that remain for months or even years. The reasons for these rare reports of long-lasting impairment are not fully understood.

Because of the possible problems with confusion and memory, it is important that I not make any important personal or business decisions during the ECT course or immediately following the course. This may mean postponing decisions regarding financial or family matters. After the treatment course, I will begin a "convalescence period," usually one to three weeks, but which varies from patient to patient. During this period I should refrain from driving, transacting business, or other activities for which impairment of memory may be problematic, until so advised by my doctor.

The conduct of ECT at this facility is under the direction of Dr. _____. I may contact him/her at (phone number: _____) if I have further questions.

I understand that I should feel free to ask questions about ECT at this time or at any time during the ECT course or thereafter from my doctor or from any other member of the ECT treatment team. I also understand that my decision to agree to ECT is being made on a voluntary basis, and that I may withdraw my consent and have the treatments stopped at any time.

I have been given a copy of this consent form to keep.

Patient:

_____   _____
Date   Signature

Person Obtaining Consent:

_____   _____
Date   Signature

Sample Patient Information Sheet

Electroconvulsive Therapy

Electroconvulsive therapy (ECT) is a safe and effective treatment for certain psychiatric disorders. ECT is most commonly used to treat patients with severe depression. It is often the safest, fastest, and most effective treatment available for this illness. ECT is also sometimes used in the treatment of patients with manic illness and patients with schizophrenia.

Treatment for depression has improved remarkably over the past 25 years. The techniques of administering ECT have also improved considerably since its introduction. During ECT, a small amount of electrical current is sent to the brain. This current induces a seizure that affects the entire brain, including the parts that control mood, appetite, and sleep. ECT is believed to correct biochemical abnormalities that underlie severe depressive illness. We know that ECT works: 80% to 90% of depressed people who receive it respond favorably, making it the most effective treatment for severe depression.

Your physician suggests that you be treated with ECT because you have a disorder that (s)he believes will respond to ECT. Discuss this with your doctor. Before ECT begins, your medical condition will be carefully assessed with a complete medical history, physical examination and laboratory tests including blood tests and an electrocardiogram (ECG).

ECT is given as a course of treatments. The number needed to successfully treat a severe depression ranges from 4 to 20. The treatments are usually given 3 times a week—Monday, Wednesday, and Friday. You must not eat or drink anything after midnight prior to your scheduled treatment. If you smoke, please try to refrain from smoking on the morning prior to your treatment.

Before your receive the treatment, a needle will be injected into a vein so that medications can be given. Although you will be asleep during the treatment, it is necessary to begin to prepare you while you are still awake. Electrodes are placed on your head for recording your EEG (electroencephalogram or brain waves). Electrodes are placed on your chest for monitoring your ECG (cardiogram or heart rhythm). A blood pressure cuff is wrapped around your wrist or ankle for monitoring your blood pressure during the treatment. When everything is connected, the ECT machine is tested to ensure that it is set properly for you.

Next, a medicine (such as methohexital) is injected that will cause you to sleep for 5 to 10 minutes. When you are asleep, a muscle relaxant (succinylcholine) is injected. This will prevent you from moving about during the treatment. It may give you a mild amount of muscle soreness after the treatment, but this soreness will pass. During this time, when you are completely asleep and your muscles are completely relaxed, the treatment is given. If you were watching the treatment instead of receiving it, you might notice your toes wiggling—but little else. You continue to receive oxygen until you awaken. Because you will be asleep, you will experience no pain during the treatment and will not feel the current or the seizure.

When you awaken, you may experience some confusion. This is partially due to the anesthesia and partially due to the treatment. With most people the confusion passes within an hour. You may have a headache the day of the treatment. It is usually helped by a pain reliever, if necessary. Other side effects, such as nausea, last for a few hours at most and are relatively uncommon. In patients with pre-existing heart disease, there is an increased risk of complications. Monitoring of heart function and other precautions, including use of additional medications if required, will be used to ensure a safe treatment.

You may experience some memory loss following the completion of the treatments. This memory loss should gradually reverse itself over the course of several weeks, but you may never remember many things that happened to you during, shortly prior to, or soon following your hospitalization and illness. Please use your memory: read, ask questions, watch continuing stories on TV. This is the best way for you to help your memory return. Because of the short-lived side effects of the treatment, it is important that you postpone any major decisions until a week or two after the ECT course.

ECT is an extremely effective form of treatment. It is often safer and more effective than available medications for the treatment of depression. It is surely safer than no treatment at all. If you have any questions about ECT, please discuss them with your doctor.

You may also wish to read the following book. It was written by a psychologist who was against people having ECT—until he had a severe depression and needed the treatment himself. His book, which describes his illness and also the experience of having ECT, is often reassuring to people who read it: *Holiday of Darkness,* by Norman S. Endler (1982: New York, Wiley-Interscience). You may also wish to read one of the following articles. They discuss why ECT is used, what is known about how ECT works, and why this treatment has been controversial: 1) "The Case for ECT," by Harold A. Sackeim (*Psychology Today,* June 1985, Volume 19, pp 36–40) and 2) "Out of the Blue: The Rehabilitation of Electroconvulsive Therapy," by Richard Abrams (*The Sciences,* November/December 1989, pp 25–30).

Appendix C

Educational Materials on ECT for Mental Health Professionals and the Public

MATERIALS FOR PROFESSIONALS

General Reading

Abrams R: Electroconvulsive Therapy. New York, Oxford University Press, 1988

American Psychiatric Association: Electroconvulsive Therapy. Task Force Report No. 14, Washington DC, American Psychiatric Association, 1978

Consensus Conference: Electroconvulsive therapy. JAMA 254:2103–2108, 1985

Endler NS, Persad E: Electroconvulsive Therapy: The Myths and the Realities. Toronto, Canada, Hans Huber, 1988

Fink M: Convulsive Therapy: Theory and Practice. New York, Raven Press, 1979

Glenn MD, Weiner RD: Electroconvulsive Therapy: A Programmed Text. Washington, DC, American Psychiatric Press, 1985

Pippard J, Ellam L: Electroconvulsive Treatment in Great Britain, 1980. London, Gaskell, 1981

Rose R, Pincus H (eds): Electroconvulsive Therapy, in American Psychiatric Press Review of Psychiatry, Vol 7. Edited by Frances AJ, Hales RE. Washington, DC, American Psychiatric Press, 1988, pp 431–532

Royal College of Psychiatrists: The Practical Administration of Electroconvulsive Therapy (ECT). London, Gaskell, 1989

Weiner RD: Does electroconvulsive therapy cause brain damage? The Behavioral and Brain Sciences 7:1–54, 1984

Theories of ECT

Fink M, Kety S, McGaugh J, Williams T (eds): Psychobiology of
Convulsive Therapy. New York, Winston-Wiley, 1974
Lerer B, Weiner RD, Belmaker RH: ECT: Basic Mechanisms. Lon-
don, John Libbey, 1984 [paperback reprint edition available
from the American Psychiatric Press]
Malitz S, Sackeim H (eds): Electroconvulsive Therapy: Clinical and
Basic Research Issues. New York, New York Academy of Sci-
ences, 1986
Sackeim HA (ed): Mechanisms of action. Convulsive Therapy
5:207–310, 1989
[See also Fink 1979 and Rose and Pincus 1988 in previous section]

Journals

Articles on electroconvulsive therapy appear throughout the
psychiatric literature, with many articles appearing in *Biological
Psychiatry*, *The American Journal of Psychiatry*, *The British Journal of
Psychiatry*, and *The Journal of Clinical Psychiatry*.

One journal is dedicated to articles on ECT: *Convulsive Therapy*
(New York, Raven Press, since 1985).

Videotapes

Fink M: Informed ECT for Health Professionals. Lake Bluff, Ill,
Somatics Inc, 1986 [25 minutes, VHS or Beta]
Healthcare Information Network: Mind and Body: Electroconvul-
sive Therapy. A New Age, A New Understanding. Portland,
Ore, MECTA Corporation, 1987 [40 minutes, VHS]

MATERIALS FOR PATIENTS
AND THEIR FAMILIES

Books

Endler NS: Holiday of Darkness: A Psychologist's Personal Journey Out of His Depression. New York, Wiley-Interscience, 1982

The following books are also easily understood by the knowledgeable layman:

Abrams R: Electroconvulsive Therapy. New York, Oxford University Press, 1988
Endler N, Persad E: Electroconvulsive Therapy: The Myths and the Realities. Toronto, H. Huber, 1988

Articles and Pamphlets

Abrams R: Out of the blue: the rehabilitation of electroconvulsive therapy. The Sciences, November/December 1989, pp 25–30
Abrams R, Swartz C: What You Need to Know About Electroconvulsive Therapy. Lake Bluff, Ill, Somatics Inc, 1988, 8 pp
Grunhaus L: Electroconvulsive Therapy: E.C.T. The Treatment, The Questions, The Answers. Ann Arbor, Mich, University of Michigan Medical Center, 1988, 9 pp [distributed by MECTA Corporation]
Sackeim HA: The case for ECT. Psychology Today, June 1985, pp 36–40

Videotapes

Fink M: Informed ECT for Health Professionals. Lake Bluff, Ill, Somatics Inc, 1986 [25 minutes, VHS or Beta]
Grunhaus L: Electroconvulsive Therapy: E.C.T. The Treatment, The Questions, The Answers. Ann Arbor, Mich, University of Michigan Medical Center, 1988 [16 minutes, VHS; distributed by MECTA Corporation]

CONTINUING EDUCATION COURSES

FOR PSYCHIATRISTS

Duke University

Visiting Fellowship: 5-day course for one or two students, designed to provide advanced training and skills in modern ECT administration. 40 CME credits.
Mini-Course: 1.5 day course designed to enable practicing clinicians to upgrade their skills in ECT. 9 CME credits.
Director: C. Edward Coffey, M.D. 919-684-5673

SUNY at Stony Brook

5-day course for four to six students, designed to provide advanced training and skills in modern ECT. 27 CME credits.
Director: Max Fink, M.D. 516-444-2929

American Psychiatric Association

At annual meetings of the APA, one-day courses are usually presented for classes of students up to 125. These are lecture/demonstrations and aim to provide discussions of such topics as treating the high-risk patient, technical aspects of treatment, and theories of ECT action. For details, see annual course offerings of APA.

Individual preceptorships

From time to time, other experienced clinicians accept visitors for varying lengths of stay at their clinics.

FOR NURSES

Courses for nurses are available at both Duke University and SUNY at Stony Brook. For information, contact Martha Cress, R.N., or Dr. Edward Coffey at Duke University, or Dr. Max Fink at SUNY at Stony Brook.

FOR ANESTHESIOLOGISTS

The courses for psychiatrists at SUNY at Stony Brook include special sessions for anesthesiologists.

Appendix D

Addresses of Present ECT Device Manufacturers in the United States and Major Characteristics of Models Offered as of February 1990

The present devices of these manufacturers meet the recommended standards of the APA Task Force on Electroconvulsive Therapy. In addition, the manufacturers distribute educational materials (books and videotapes), which are useful in learning about ECT.

ELCOT Sales, Inc.
14 East 60th Street
New York, NY 10022
212-688-0900

MECTA Corp.
7015 S.W. McEwan Road
Lake Oswego, OR 97035
503-624-8778

Medcraft
433 Boston Post Road
Darien, CT 06820
800-638-2896

Somatics, Inc.
910 Sherwood Drive
Unit 17
Lake Bluff, IL 60044
800-642-6761

Table 2. Major characteristics of ECT devices available in the
United States as of February 1990

Manufacturer, model	Waveform	Mode	Built-in impedance self-test	EEG monitoring
ELCOT MF-1000	Pulse Sine wave	Constant current Constant voltage Constant energy[*]	Yes	Yes
MECTA SR-1,2 MECTA JR-1,2	Pulse	Constant current	Yes	SR-1,2
Medcraft B25 Medcraft B24	Pulse Sine wave	Constant energy[*] Constant voltage	No[**] No	No No
Somatics Thymatron-DG	Pulse	Constant current	Yes	Yes

[*]With the Elcot MF-1000, the constant energy option may be achieved with either constant current or constant voltage principles. With the Medcraft B25, the constant energy stimulus level is achieved by constant current principles.
[**]Incorporates sensing circuitry to automatically terminate stimulus if impedance during delivery of current is too high or low.

Appendix E

Responsibilities for Local Facilities Regarding ECT

1. The director of each facility, or his or her designee, should appoint an individual responsible for maintaining up-to-date policies and procedures regarding ECT and for seeing that they are met (Section 7.1).
2. Each facility should stipulate the components of a pre-ECT evaluation (Sections 9, 6, and 13.3.4).
3. Local policies and procedures for the administration of ECT should be developed, including issues related to anesthesia; stimulus electrode placement; stimulus dosing; physiological monitoring; management of missed, inadequate, or prolonged seizures; frequency and number of treatments to be administered; and use of outpatient ECT (Section 11).
4. Each facility should specify the characteristics of an abortive or inadequate seizure and a policy regarding restimulation (Sections 11.8.1 and 11.8.2).
5. Each facility should have policies to abort prolonged seizures (Sections 4.5 and 11.8.4).
6. Each facility should be prepared to manage cardiovascular complications associated with ECT. (Sections 4.3, 7, and 8).
7. Each facility should develop a policy regarding the number of treatments at which a formal assessment of the need for continued ECT is required (Sections 5.3, 11.10.2, and 13.3).
8. Facilities providing multiple monitored ECT (MMECT) should specify treatment procedures including intervals between seizures and between sessions, the recommended and maximum number of seizures per session, and the delivery of anesthesia and muscle relaxation, as well as information provided to the consentor comparing benefits and risks of MMECT as compared to standard ECT (Section 11.11).
9. Facilities administering ECT to pregnant women should assure that ready access to means of managing fetal emergencies is present (Section 6.3).

10. Each facility should assure that qualified personnel test new ECT devices prior to their first use (Section 11.4.2).

11. Biomedical electronics personnel should be consulted prior to the use of external monitoring devices to assure electrical safety (Section 11.7.1).

12. Local requirements pertaining to standards and intervals of testing for electrical safety of medical devices involving patient contact should be ascertained and followed (Section 11.4.2).

13. Each facility should assure that the treatment area provides a single electrical supply circuit for all electrical treatment and monitoring devices in contact with the patient (Sections 11.4.3 and 11.7.1).

14. Each facility should develop policies and procedures to assure proper informed consent for adults, minors, and those lacking capacity to consent. Procedures should be included for anesthesia consent, if required by local policy. All consent policies and procedures should be consistent with state and local regulatory requirements, including those applicable to emergency situations (Section 5).

15. Each facility should develop a written consent document (a summary of general information related to ECT to provide to the consentor may also be helpful) (Section 5.4 and Appendix B).

16. Facilities providing outpatient ECT should monitor adherence to relevant policies and procedures, including patient selection and treatment technique (Section 11.12).

17. Each facility providing outpatient ECT is encouraged to provide a written instruction sheet to patients regarding behavioral limitations (Section 11.12.3).

18. Each facility using continuation/maintenance ECT should devise procedures for pre-ECT evaluation in such cases (Section 13.3.4).

19. Each facility should assure that adequate documentation regarding ECT is carried out (Section 14).

20. Each facility should implement a quality assurance program to monitor adherence to policies, detect occurrences of major adverse effects, and correct observed insufficiencies (Section 7.1).

21. Each facility should develop a formal written plan for the provision and maintenance of ECT privileges (Section 16.2). This plan should include means to establish that practitioners have received adequate training and have demonstrated clinical competency (Sections 7, 15, and 16.1).

22. Each member of the ECT treatment team should be clinically privileged to practice in his or her respective ECT-related duties (Sections 7 and 16).
23. Each facility should determine which individuals under what circumstances may serve as anesthetists for ECT (Sections 7.2.2. and 16).
24. Each facility should determine the level of attendance required at ECT-related continuing education programs for privileging purposes (Sections 15.7.1 and 16).

Appendix F

Major Topics Covered in Recommendations Section

Index